2 Frontiers in European Radiology

Editors-in-Chief

A.L. Baert · E. Boijsen
W.A. Fuchs · F.H.W. Heuck

Editorial Board

P. Bodart · G. Breitling · L. Dalla-Palma · W. Dihlmann
G. du Boulay · P. Edholm · C. Fauré · H. Frommhold
W. Frommhold · T. Greitz · V. Hegedüs · H. Kaufmann
E. Koivisto · L. Kreel · M. Laval-Jeantet · A. Lunderquist
J.H. Middlemiss · I. Obrez · F. Pinet · H. Pokieser · J. Remy
P. Rossi · T. Sherwood · A. Wackenheim · F. Weill

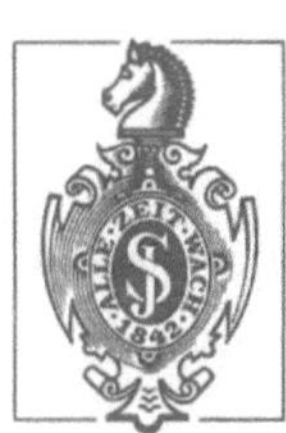

Springer-Verlag
Berlin Heidelberg New York 1982

Professor Dr. Albert L. Baert

Universitaire Ziekenhuizen, Department of Diagnostic Radiology,
Capucijnenvoer 35, B-3000 Leuven

Professor Dr. Erik Boijsen

University Hospital, Department of Diagnostic Radiology, S-22185 Lund

Professor Dr. Walter A. Fuchs

Inselspital Bern, Institut für Diagnostische Radiologie der Universität,
CH-3010 Bern

Professor Dr. Friedrich H. W. Heuck

Radiologisches Institut im Zentrum Radiologie, Katharinenhospital
(Lehrkrankenhaus der Universität Tübingen),
Kriegsbergstr. 60, D-7000 Stuttgart

With 70 Figures (in 84 Separate Illustrations)

ISBN-13: 978-3-642-48324-0   e-ISBN-13: 978-3-642-48322-6
DOI: 10.1007/978-3-642-48322-6

Typesetting, printing and bookbinding: Konrad Triltsch, Würzburg
2121/3130-543210

Preface

The second volume of *Frontiers in European Radiology* covers two very promising techniques in diagnostic radiology, namely digital radiography and nuclear magnetic resonance imaging. Leading experts in both fields from Europe and the United States were invited to give a critical overview; digital fluoroscopy is reported on mainly by American scientists since this technique has been developed primarily in the United States, while the results of nuclear magnetic resonance imaging are presented by British groups currently at the forefront of research in this field. The papers reflect the state of the art at mid-1981, when the contributors gathered for the yearly symposium on Current Topics in Diagnostic Radiology in Berne, Switzerland.

Nuclear magnetic resonance imaging, also known as spin imaging or zeugmatography, has produced striking progress within the past few years – even within the past few months – as described in three papers of this volume. The images generally reflect the distribution of mobile protons contained within water and fats, and provide remarkable discrimination between different tissues. Malignant tissue might be identified with this technique, and a wide range of disorders associated with water concentration, diffusion, and flow would be amenable to study; the measurement of blood flow could be particularly interesting.

It would be extremely useful to combine the spin-imaging method with topical nuclear magnetic resonance spectroscopy in order to evaluate the metabolic states of different tissues. However, it should be noted that the metabolites P-31 and C-12 have typical concentrations of about 1–5 mM, whereas the protons are present at concentrations of up to about 100 mM. Acceptable signal-to-noise ratios could be obtained only at the expense of a substantial reduction in spatial resolution, and yet there are high hopes that the enormous technical problems faced will be overcome. A first step in this direction might be the use of other currently available imaging methods such as computerized tomography and sonography for topographical localization, in combination with surface coils or topical NMR using large-bore, high-resolution magnets.

Digital radiography, i.e., photoelectronic imaging, is currently challenging conventional radiological imaging which uses photographic film. Digital subtraction fluoroscopy and fluorography, computerized tomography, computerized radiography, sonography, and nuclear magnetic resonance imaging all produce photoelectronic information which may be processed, stored, and displayed by means of a specialized image-computer with a large-capacity digital memory using magnetic discs.

Image processing, such as edge enhancement, subtraction, measurements of size, volume, density, and number, pattern recognition, and time parameters, will then become possible by the formulation of adequate computer programs. However, reproduction of images for clinical work and archival storage will still be based on film recording – preferably 10×10 cm images – owing to the logistic problems which diagnostic radiology departments will continue to face. Most important are the high costs involved in the organization of a photoelectronic archival storage and transmission system to serve clinical wards. Moreover, such a system might remove control and diagnostic evaluation of radiological investigations from the sphere of the radiology department.

Digital subtraction angiography is already an established method for demonstrating morphological vascular abnormalities in the head and neck arteries, the abdominal aorta, the renal arteries, and the peripheral arterial vessels. However, the full potential of the method, particularly with regard to the evaluation of myocardial function and flow measurements by densitometry, has still not been clearly defined by technological progress.

April 1982   W. A. Fuchs

Contents

NMR as an Imaging Method

W. Loeffler[1]

1 Introduction

In principle, all fields or particles which have the following characteristics are suitable for medical imaging:

First, they must interact with the body tissue, secondly, it must still be possible for them to penetrate through the body to an adequate degree and, thirdly, a spatial coordination of this interaction must be possible.

The fact that x-rays, even 80 years after their discovery, still play the dominant role makes it evident how difficult it is to achieve a simultaneous fulfilment of these three conditions. The inadequate penetration depth of electromagnetic radiation of greater wavelength into the body is one reason for this. Throughout the total spectral range, beginning with soft x-rays and proceeding over ultraviolet and visible light as far as microwaves, the strong attenuation of the radiation in the body prevents an application for imaging. Only at still greater wave lengths, that is to say, in the short-wave range, does the penetration depth of the field into the body increase again.

If an attempt is made to use electromagnetic fields from this range, the following difficulty arises. An adequate penetration depth is only attained with wave lengths greater than approximately 20 cm. But in this wave length range, with quasi-optical methods of imaging, it is no longer possible to attain the necessary spatial resolution. For, as is known for example from the optical microscope with such a system, the limit of resolution is of the same order of magnitude as the wave length used. If, in spite of this, it is intended to use this part of the electromagnetic spectrum for image production, other than quasi-optical methods must be applied

---

1 Siemens AG, Unternehmensbereich Medizinische Technik, Henkestraße 127,
  D-8520 Erlangen

for image production and these methods are somewhat less obvious. Nuclear magnetic resonance imaging represents such a method.

Although the effect of nuclear magnetic resonance (NMR) was already known in the middle of the 1940s, the first proposals for its application in imaging, especially in respect of human beings, are only 8–10 years old (*Damadian* 1971; *Lauterbur* 1973).

As a consequence, first of all, some general, fundamental concepts from the field of NMR are explained, before going on to show in detail how it is possible to apply this effect in producing images.

2 NMR

All atomic nuclei with an uneven number of protons or neutrons, that is to say, about two-thirds of all stable atomic nuclei, possess an angular momentum or spin. Since all atomic nuclei are electrically charged, a magnetic moment is associated with the angular momentum, similar to a circular current causing a magnetic field as shown in Fig. 1. With certain limitations, which will be explained later, it can be said that these nuclei behave similarly to rotating magnetic gyroscopes. The simplest and, at the same time, most abundant nucleus of this kind in the human body is the hydrogen nucleus, the proton.

Figure 2 and 3 show the behavior of an assembly of such atomic nuclei on being subjected to an external magnetic field. If the field-free case shown in the upper part of Fig. 2 is first considered, the alignment of the nuclear magnetic moments will be arbitrary. The probability of the nuclei orientating themselves in a given direction is equal for all directions. On applying a field, it is different. This sets a direction in space in relation to which the nuclear moments can align. It can now be shown that on the grounds of quantum mechanics, for protons only two positioning possibilities exist; one parallel to the field and one antiparallel to the

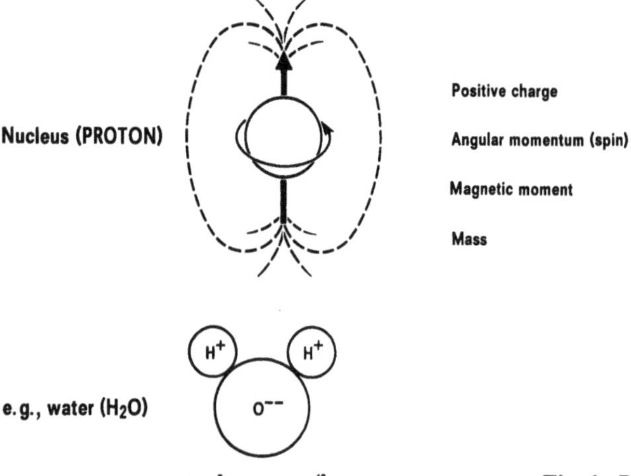

Fig. 1. Physical characterization of nuclei

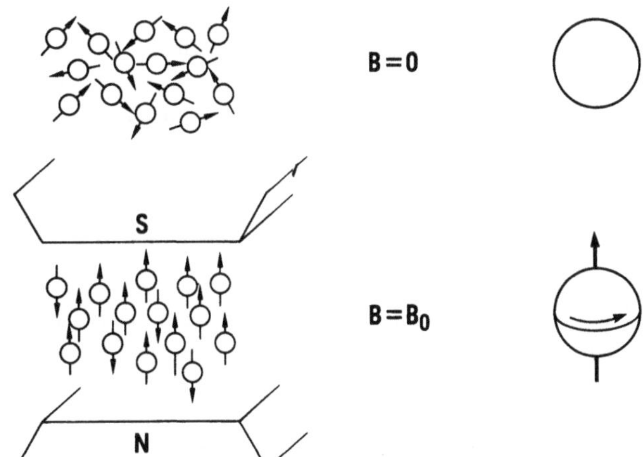

Fig. 2. Formation of
nuclear magnetization

field. Actually, more nuclei align themselves parallel to the field, because, for reasons of energy, this is more favorable. If a large number of atomic nuclei is now considered, then because of this preponderance of nuclear moments aligned parallel to the field, an externally detectable, macroscopic magnetic moment associated with a macroscopic angular momentum arises in the magnetic field. It is then said that the specimen, a water drop for example, is magnetized in the field, and the extent of the magnetization is represented by the magnetic moment per volume, that is to say, in this case, by the preponderant number of nuclei aligned parallel to the field. The magnetization which arises as an average value over many atomic nuclei behaves, in fact, just as one would expect a magnetic gyroscope to behave.

In Fig. 3 the movement of the magnetization in the field is represented symbolically with the aid of a rotating sphere. In the same way as a compass needle, the magnetization aligns parallel to the field in a state of equilibrium. If the magne-

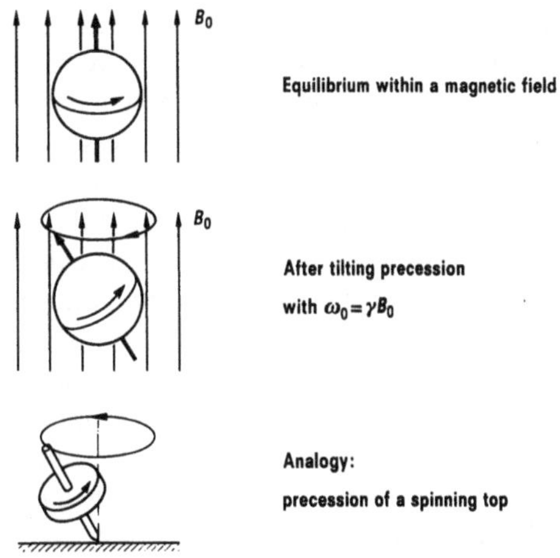

Fig. 3. Precession

tization is then deflected out of this direction, it endeavors to return to the old, energy favorable position. However, this is prevented by the angular momentum, exactly as in the case of a rotating gyroscope, which in spite of the influence of gravity cannot fall over. The resulting movement is called precession. The angular frequency ω_0 of the precession of the nuclear magnetization about the field direction is proportional to the strength of the magnetic field B_0 :

$$\omega_0 = \gamma \cdot B_0$$

The constant γ is called the gyromagnetic ratio and is a characteristic of the atomic nuclei concerned. For protons in a field of 0.1 T, that is, in the old units 1 kGauss, this rotation or precessional frequency is 4.26 MHz. To detect the precession of the nuclear magnetization the specimen is surrounded by a coil in which an alternating current of the same frequency is induced.

To tilt the magnetization out of its equilibrium state parallel to the magnetic field and thus induce the precession, a small alternating magnetic field is created perpendicular to the static field, by transmitting an alternating current pulse through the measuring coil. If the frequency of this alternating magnetic field synchronizes exactly with the precessional frequency of the nuclear magnetization, then this turns out of its state of equilibrium, even if the strength of the alternating field is much smaller than that of the static field. After the magnetization has turned through an angle of preferably 90° the radio frequency (rf) alternating field is switched off, and the apparatus is switched over to a receiving mode so that it can subsequently detect the voltage induced in the coil by the precessing magnetization. Instead of the sine-shaped NMR signal, it is possible to plot its frequency spectrum. Both representations are equivalent and can be converted from one to the other by a Fourier transform.

If the atomic nuclei, whose resonance is being observed, exist in various chemical compounds, in an NMR experiment not just one single resonance line is obtained which corresponds to a single resonance frequency, but instead a number of lines are obtained which lie close together. The intensity ratio of these lines represents exactly the abundance ratio with which the element concerned is to be found in the various compounds. Then, for example, with the aid of the ^{31}P-NMR, it is possible to measure the relative concentration of ATP, phosphocreatine, and inorganic phosphate. In recent years, these experiments have been successfully transferred from the test tube, where naturally the same result can be obtained by conventional analytic means at less expense, to intact biologic tissue (*Gordon* et al. 1980). Thus, with small laboratory animals, as well as in human extremities, it was possible to demonstrate that with ^{31}P-NMR, the metabolic condition and degree of fatigue of muscular tissue can be examined.

Because of the relatively low concentration of phosphorus in body tissue, these measurements demand a powerful magnetic field with the corresponding technical outlay. Even then, this low concentration of phosphorus excludes the possibility of producing an image of the phosphorus distribution in the body with the same resolution, as is the case with the much more frequently occurring protons. It is rather that these measurements always represent an average value obtained from selected volume locations, whereby on grounds of sensitivity the size of these areas, in the case of small laboratory animals or in the body close to the surface, is at least a few cm^3, and at greater depths in the body even becomes 100 cm^3.

3 Relaxation

The precession of the nuclear magnetization in an experiment of the type described decays with time. The corresponding attenuation process is called relaxation.

A distinction must be made between two processes which proceed simultaneously, but which are described by two different time constants which can naturally also be measured separately. By way of explanation, it is possible to think of the precessing vector of magnetization as being composed of two components, a stationary component in the direction of the magnetic field and a second component rotating in a plane at right angles to this. Now on the one hand, there is a tendency to reach the initial value of thermal equilibrium again, that is the situation where the magnetization is parallel to the field. This process is called longitudinal relaxation or, since the interaction of the nuclei with the surrounding lattice is responsible for it, spin-lattice relaxation. The corresponding time constant is generally denoted by T_1. On the other hand, the size of the rotating transverse component reduces with a generally shorter time constant T_2, because of an interaction of the nuclei between each other. Therefore, this process is called transverse or spin-spin relaxation. These processes have the effect that after a time the magnetization is turned back to its initial position, parallel to the magnetic field, so that no further precession is detectable.

This simple model with two time constants and exponential time behavior describes the relaxation of the nuclear magnetization in homogeneous liquids quite well. However, in rigid bodies the decay of the transverse magnetization is very rapid and not exponential, so that such a description is no longer valid. In its consistency, biologic tissue lies between liquids and solids. Besides this, it is normally inhomogeneous in the physical and chemical sense. It is frequently necessary to describe the relaxation behavior by means of a sum of several exponential functions with various time constants (*Weisman* et al. 1981). If in this case only an effective relaxation time is given, then this is dependent on the measuring process, and if different installations are used for measurements and different measuring procedures are applied, appropriate care must be taken to avoid misunderstandings.

4 NMR Imaging Methods

In an NMR experiment of the type described, all measured quantities are average values over the whole specimen which fills the measuring coil. In order to produce an image, it is necessary to make the contributions to the NMR signal from the various regions of the specimen distinguishable. For this purpose, various procedures have been developed which, however, all rely on the same basic principle.

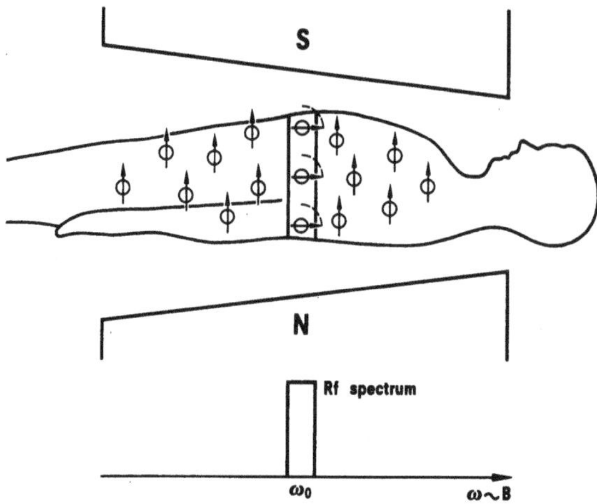

Fig. 4. Selective excitation of a slice

The strength of the static magnetic field is made spatially dependent in a specific manner. Because of the proportionality between the NMR frequency and the magnetic field strength, it is then possible to ascribe the various contributions to the NMR signal to the location in which they arise by means of a frequency analysis.

A simple way of providing the magnetic field with the required locational dependency is either by means of suitably shaping the pole caps of a magnet, or by an appropriate arrangement of current carrying coils which ensure that the magnetic field strength varies linearly as a function of the location. It is said of such a field that it has a linear gradient where the direction of this field gradient is defined as the direction of the field change. For NMR imaging air-core coil arrangements are used in order to change the direction of the field gradients as quickly as possible. Nevertheless, in the following illustrations, for the sake of clarity, a field gradient is symbolized by means of inclined pole caps.

Figure 4 shows the selection of a slice in the body for imaging with the aid of such a field dependence. As already mentioned, the precessional frequency of the magnetization is proportional to the magnetic field strength. Thus, here, the NMR frequency also varies with the magnetic field along the longitudinal axis of the body. If one thinks in terms of a row of parallel axial planes through the body, then the resonance frequency within each plane is the same, but it alters from one plane to the next. To tilt the magnetization out of its equilibrium state parallel to the field, in order to start the precession, it is necessary to generate an alternating rf magnetic field whose frequency synchronizes exactly with the precession frequency. This means that in the case shown in Fig. 4 the magnetization is induced to precess in only one single plane. All other regions remain uninfluenced by this excitation pulse, and therefore cannot contribute subsequently to the NMR signal. This mode of slice selection is known as selective excitation (*Garroway* et al. 1974).

Figure 5 demonstrates how an image can be obtained from a slice selected in this manner. To do this, after excitation the direction of the magnetic field gradient is turned into a perpendicular plane as shown in Fig. 5. The magnetization which has been induced to process is now influenced by a magnetic field of varying

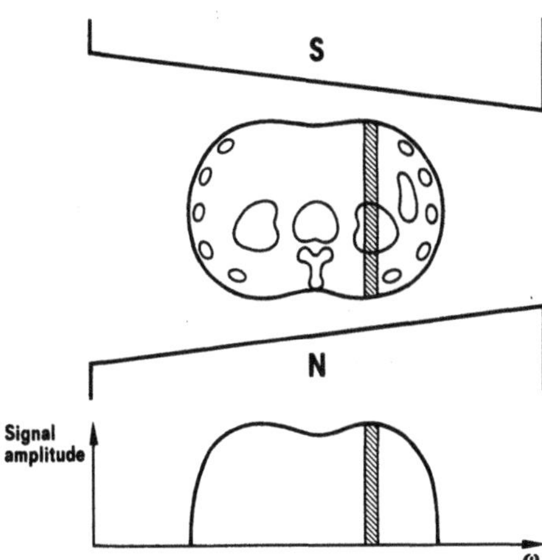

Fig. 5. Recording of a projection
in a linear field gradient

strengths, according to whether it is further to the left, in the region of lesser field
strength, or further to the right, in the region of higher field strength. As already
mentioned, the corresponding precession frequency varies over the slice in the same
way as the field strength. Thus, in a coil which surrounds the body, a signal is
received which contains all the NMR frequencies arising. However, if the spectrum
of this signal is analyzed, as shown below in Fig. 5, it can be seen that again simple
relationships exist. All atomic nuclei in a strip perpendicular to the direction of the
gradient are subjected to the same magnetic field, and therefore contribute with the
same frequency to the total signal. Thus, at the corresponding position in the spectrum, an intensity will be received which is exactly proportional to the number of
nuclei in such a strip. Naturally, this applies to every possible strip through the
object perpendicular to the direction of the field gradient. In other words, this
frequency spectrum represents a projection of the proton density within the slice,
onto the direction of the field gradient (*Lauterbur* 1973).

It is now possible to proceed as in computerized tomography. The same
measurement is repeated for other directions of the gradient. From these projections, an image of the slice is reconstructed by using exactly the same algorithm as
in CT.

But, as opposed to x-ray CT in NMR tomography, alternative procedures to
create images are possible. On the one hand, there are the so-called planar procedures which have the characteristic that the NMR signal is always simultaneously
registered from the whole excited slice resulting, for example, in the exposure of
projections. Besides this, there are also procedures for scanning a slice point by
point (*Damadian* et al. 1978) or line by line (*Mansfield* and *Maudsley* 1977), as well
as three-dimensional reconstruction procedures (*Lauterbur* et al. 1980), in which
the NMR signal from the whole object, that is to say, from all the slices which are
being examined, is recorded simultaneously. As opposed to the planar procedures,
these last-named procedures have a sensitivity advantage. However, they also have
the disadvantage that it is necessary to wait until the end of the complete
examination, before the first sectional images can be reconstructed. An error in the
setting or in the positioning thus requires the tiresome repetition of the complete

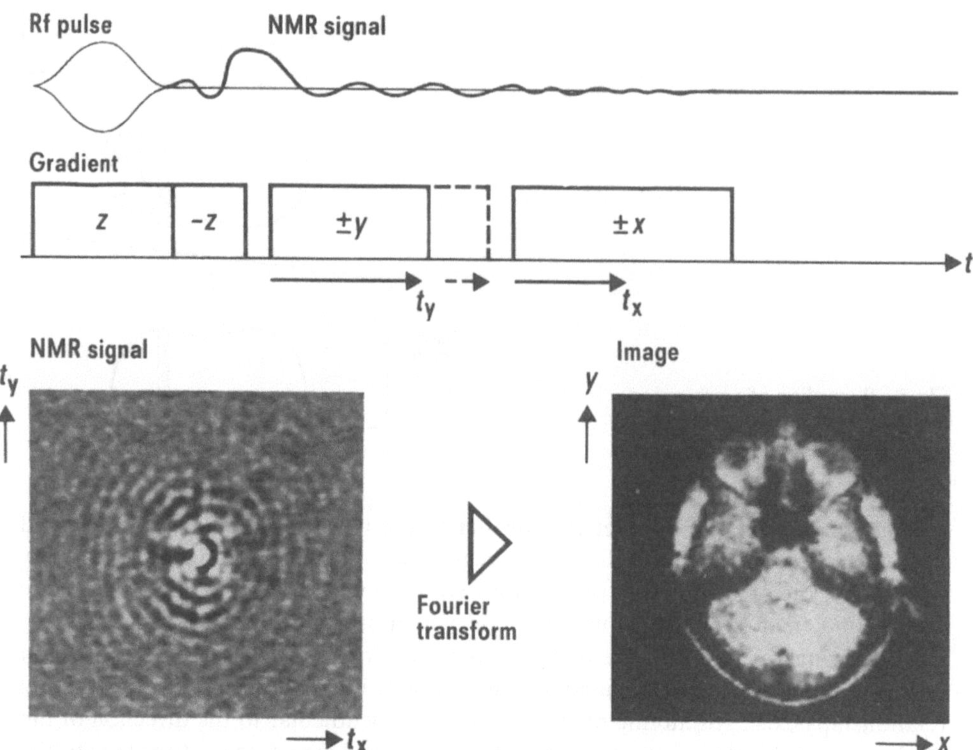

Fig. 6. Two-dimensional Fourier Tomography (*Kumar* et al. 1975)

measuring procedure, whereas in the planar procedures, after the exposure of each individual slice, the corresponding image can be immediately reconstructed. The same argument applies in the case of movement artefacts. Also in this case, with a three-dimensional procedure, the whole examination must be repeated and not just one slice.

Figure 6 shows the scheme of an alternative planar image formation procedure. The selection of a slice by imposing a selective rf pulse, with the field gradient switched on, proceeds in the same manner as already explained. In the subsequent measuring sequence for producing an image, no rotated field gradients are used as when reconstructing from projections, but two field gradients of fixed direction are used perpendicular to one another. The time sequence is as follows: After a y-gradient pulse of variable length the x-gradient is switched on, and during this the NMR signal is registered. This is to say, the slice is always projected onto the same direction, denoted here by x, and by means of the variable gradient a spatially varying phase characteristic is imprinted from scan to scan in the perpendicular direction. If the resulting data sets are arranged as the lines of a matrix corresponding to the y-gradient pulse length, an image as shown below left in Fig. 6 is obtained. It represents exactly the spatial frequency spectrum of the slice being examined and so it is only necessary to apply a two-dimensional Fourier transform in order to obtain an image of the usual type. This principle of image formation is based on a proposal by *Kumar* et al. (1975) and is called Fourier

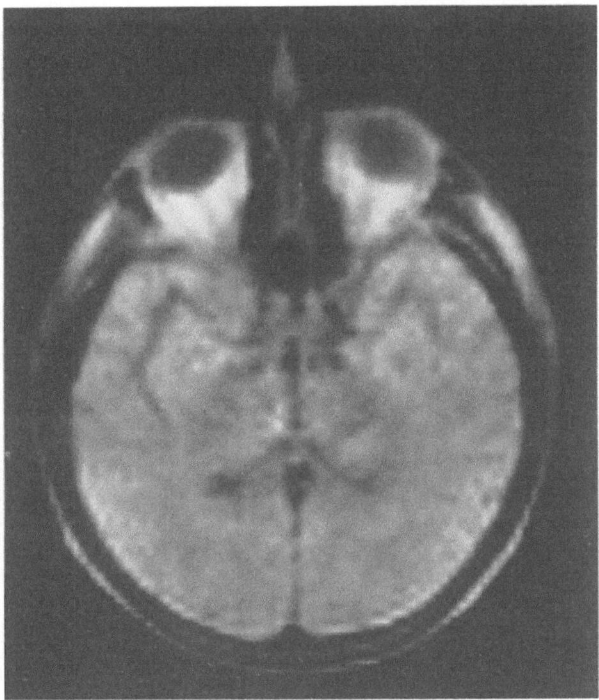

Fig. 7. Axial NMR tomogram

Zeugmatography or Fourier Tomography. In the first instance, the procedure may seem somewhat complicated, but it can be shown mathematically that it is equivalent to the backprojection algorithms known from CT. Figure 7 shows an NMR tomogram obtained by using the Fourier method.

In NMR imaging, one is by no means limited to transverse slices. As already mentioned, the magnetic field gradients which determine the position and direction of the slice are produced by the aid of current-carrying coils. By simply switching over the currents in these coils, it is thus possible to also measure coronary and sagittal slices (*Holland* et al. 1980).

The quantity shown in Fig. 7 is the amplitude of the NMR signal from the corresponding regions of the skull. Regions which are rich in protons, that is, in particular those containing much water, deliver a strong signal and appear correspondingly bright. On the other hand, bones which have a low water content appear almost as dark as the air-filled body cavities. Fat, which naturally also contains many protons, consequently appears very bright. Therefore, the images in first order approximation display the proton concentration in the corresponding regions. However, depending on the measuring sequence used, the relaxation times also contribute, to a greater or lesser degree, to the image impression.

In fact the quantitative dependence of the NMR signal S, as measured by the pulse sequence described and shown in the image, on the relaxation times T_1 and T_2 is given by the formula:

$$S = \tau\, e^{-\tau/T_2}\,(1 - e^{-T/T_1})$$

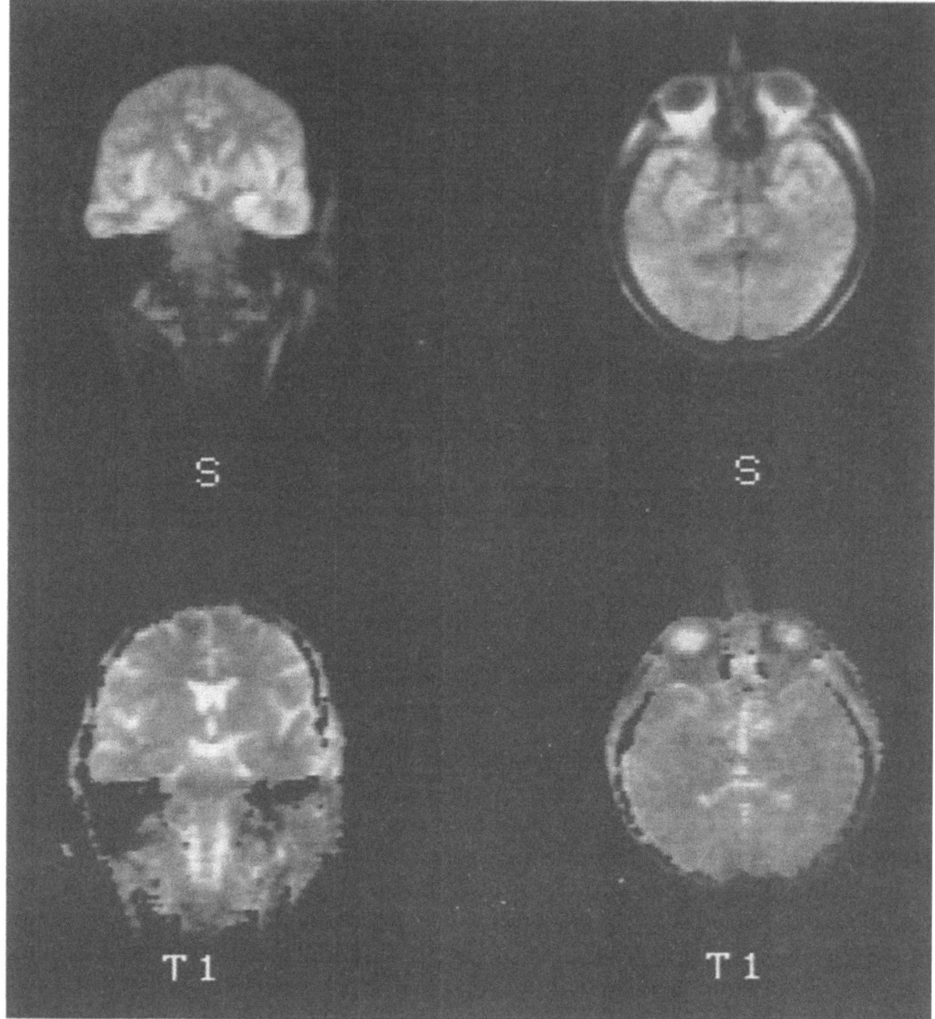

Fig. 8. Comparison of images showing the local amplitude of the NMR signal (S) with images displaying purely the longitudinal relaxation time (T_1)

T is the time interval between subsequent scans in the imaging sequence. In Fig. 7, T is about 2 s. τ is the time between the excitation of the spin system by the rf pulse and the reading of the signal. In our images, this is approximately 50 ms. Finally, ϱ is the proton concentration in the tissue. Because of the factor shown in brackets at the end, this equation demands a decrease in the NMR signal for long relaxation times T_1.

It is possible to exploit this dependence by altering the pulse repetition time T to obtain images with varying accentuation of the longitudinal relaxation time T_1. Naturally, it is also possible to influence the dependence on the transversal relaxation time T_2 by varying the time τ. It is even possible to go a step further and calculate a pure representation of T_1 or T_2 from a number of recorded images with varying T or τ, by applying normalizing procedures. In Fig. 8, such normalized representations of the longitudinal relaxation time T_1 are shown in comparison to normal images of the same slice, which represent the spatially resolved NMR signal, the quantity S.

As can be seen, NMR imaging permits the soft tissue of the body to be represented in very many different ways. In a physical sense, it is always a combination of the quantities proton density, longitudinal relaxation time T_1, and transverse relaxation time T_2. With the aid of more complicated measuring sequences and appropriate normalizing procedures, it is also possible to represent each of these three magnitudes in isolation. The future will show which type of representation provides the best diagnosis possibility. In this respect, it is quite probable that for the examination of various organs or the diagnosis of different diseases different, selectable measuring processes will be developed in order to yield the best results.

A procedure which results in images with strong accentuation of the relaxation time T_1 is the so-called inversion recovery technique. Figure 9 shows a coronary section through the skull obtained by this method. In doing this, the magnetization is first of all inverted by means of an rf pulse. Then the total magnetization will be aligned antiparallel to the magnetic field. After this, a certain time is allowed to elapse in which the magnetization approaches its equilibrium value according to

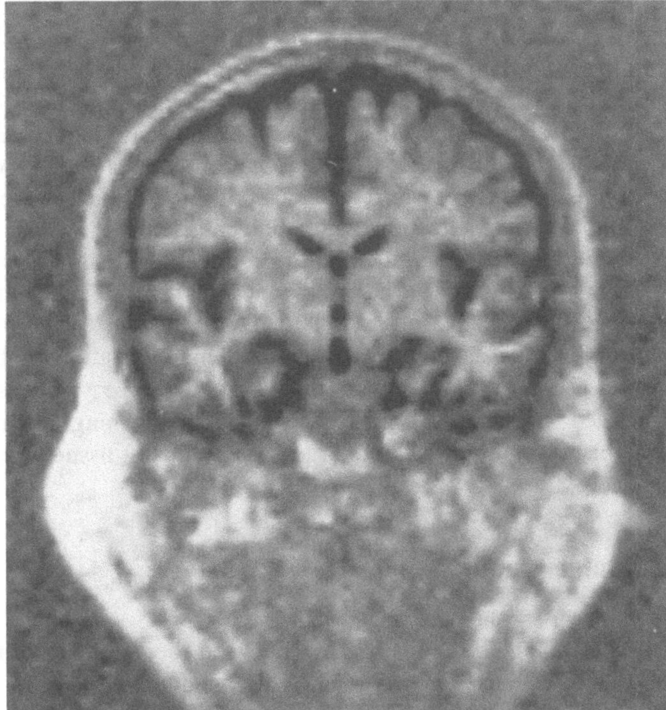

Fig. 9. Coronal section obtained with the "inversion-recovery" method

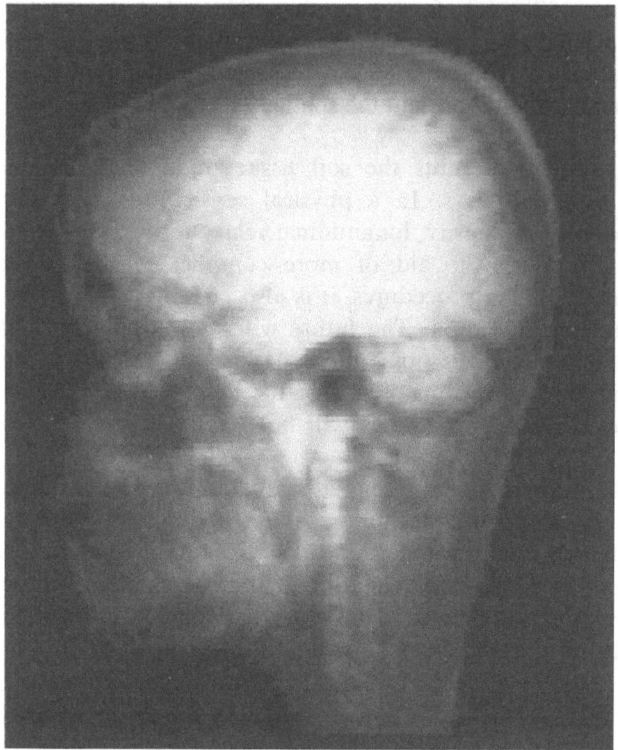

Fig. 10. Lateral NMR
projection of the head

the local spin-lattice relaxation time. Following this waiting period – typically 0.4 s – a projection is recorded in accordance with the procedure described. This has the result that the magnetization in the locations with longer relaxation times, as in the ventricles, is still inverted; these locations appear correspondingly dark, whereas locations with very short relaxation times, which have almost reached their equilibrium magnetization, are displayed bright.

Naturally, it is also possible to produce NMR images which, just as in the case of x-ray images or the survey exposures at CT installations, show projections through the object being examined. To do this, instead of the selective excitation of only one layer as described, the total magnetization in the object is excited to precess. Figure 10 shows an image of this type. Since such exposures can be obtained in the same time as normal sectional images, it is possible that they are suitable for rapidly checking large regions for soft tissue processes.

5 Image Quality

In NMR imaging the reationship between the geometry of the object to be imaged and the image itself is provided by the magnetic field gradients. Since in principle, the magnitude of these field gradients can be adjusted as desired, the sharpness or spatial resolution of the image is not subject to geometrical limitations, such as is imposed in CT by the detector aperture. Thus, if possible, artefacts are disregarded, the image quality being limited only by the noise superimposed on the image. In spite of the theoretical arbitrary adjustment of the spatial resolution, naturally, this noise results in a limitation when recognizing small objects.

On the one hand, the cause of this noise lies in the ohmic resistance of the rf receiver coil. This noise source can be minimized by appropriate modifications to the apparatus. On the other hand, the thermal movement of the electrical charge carriers in the patient himself induces noise in the apparatus. This noise is unavoidable. It would otherwise be necessary to cool the patient down almost to absolute zero.

In competition with the noise is the NMR signal from the body. This signal increases with the strength of the magnet used. Thus, the signal-to-noise ratio, which is decisive for image quality, increases approximately linearly with the strength of the magnetic field, provided that the noise from the patient himself predominates over other noise sources (*Hoult* and *Lauterbur* 1979). Thus, with an otherwise ideal apparatus, the image quality achievable is limited by the strength of the magnet used. For this reason, high magnetic fields are desirable.

On the other hand, the penetration depth of the rf magnetic field into the body decreases with increasing NMR frequency. This imposes a natural limit for the strength of the static magnetic field, which for protons is expected to lie between 0.3 and 1 T, depending on whether the body or the head is being investigated (*Bottomley* and *Andrew* 1978).

There is another simple possibility of reducing noise. The measuring procedure can be repeated a number of times and the data added. The noise is accordingly reduced at the expense of a longer total measuring time.

Nevertheless, the magnet for producing the static field in an NMR tomography installation plays a particularly important part. For field strengths up to 0.2 T, water-cooled coils of aluminium strip or copper tubes are mainly used. At this field strength, their electrical power consumption is already 55 kW. Therefore, for higher field strengths, super-conducting magnetic systems are preferable. In these, the coils are cooled down to 4.2 K, that is −269 °C, by liquid helium. The conducting material – mostly niobium alloys – loses its electrical resistance at this temperature, so that once a current is flowing it persists for a very long time, almost without loss, and thus permits high magnetic fields to be produced very economically. Indeed, replacement of the evaporating helium must be provided for which, according to the rate of vaporization, can be very expensive.

6 Potential Hazards

Before one enters such a machine or expects someone else to do so, it should naturally be ascertained that the fields applied during measurements of this kind are harmless to human beings. Therefore, here are a few words about the compatibility of magnetic fields. A distinction must be made between static magnetic fields, that is, those which remain constant in time, and dynamic magnetic fields, that is, those which change with time. So far as static fields are concerned, experience has been built up for about 30 years in nuclear physics laboratories, with large magnets for accelerators and bubble chambers. Over this period, there have been no reports on harmful effects of static fields below 0.5 T, although numerous people have been subjected to fields of such intensities, in some case, for a long time (*Budinger* 1979). Since all NMR installations for imaging with protons work in this range below 0.5 T, also in this instance no injurious effect is to be expected from the static field.

At field strengths between 0.5 and 2 T, there are conflicting reports on the biologic effects, although even here no concrete injuries to human beings or animals are spoken of, nor is the mechanism of the effects made known (*Budinger* 1979). On grounds of sensitivity, fields of this strength must be used for the metabolic examinations with ^{31}P which have already been referred to. Further examinations in the immediate future should make clear whether actual effects of the static magnetic field can be detected and, if so, from which field strengths the possibility of injury can no longer be excluded.

Magnetic fields which change with time lead to alternating electrical currents in the body, as a consequence of the laws of induction. For these types of current exactly the same loading limits apply as for currents which flow through the body due to contact with external voltage sources. For low-frequency alternating currents it is thus necessary to avoid interference with the conduction of stimuli, especially in the heart, and in the case of higher frequencies, such as are used in diathermy, care must be taken that no overheating of the tissue occurs. The NMR tomography installations at present in use lie within the safe ranges for both the effects nominated.

Beyond this, recently the results were made known of experiments on the influence of such fields as are used in NMR, on human and animal cell cultures (*Cooke* and *Morris* 1981; *Thomas* and *Morris* 1981; *Wolff* et al. 1980). In spite of the long exposure time of up to 14 h, no damage to the chromosomes or to the DNA could be confirmed. Similarly, no influence on the metabolic activity of various bacteria strains could be detected, although such cell cultures and bacteria were used which had shown themselves to be very sensitive to ionizing radiation, UV radiation, or toxic chemicals.

It is thus possible to assume with a clear conscience that even in the case of repeated examinations, no injurious effect is to be expected from the fields to which the patient is subjected during NMR imaging.

References

Bottomley PA, Andrew ER (1978) Rf-magnetic field penetration, phase shift and power dissipation in biological tissue: Implications for NMR imaging. Phys Med Biol 23:630–643
Budinger TF (1979) Thresholds for physiological effects due to rf and magnetic fields used in NMR imaging. IEEE Trans Nucl Sci NS-26:2821–2825
Cooke P, Morris PG (1981) The effects of NMR exposure on living organisms. II. A genetic study of human lymphocytes. Br J Radiol 54:622–625
Damadian R (1971) Tumor detection by nuclear magnetic resonance. Science 171:1151–1153
Damadian R, Minkoff L, Goldsmith M, Koutcher JA (1978) Field focusing nuclear magnetic resonance (FONAR). Naturwissenschaften 65:250–252

Garroway AN, Grannell PK, Mansfield P (1974) Image formation in NMR by a selective irradiative process. J Phys C 7:L 457–L 462

Gordon RE, Hanley PE, Shaw D, Gadian DG, Radda GK, Styles P, Bore PJ, Chan L (1980) Localization of metabolites in animals using ^{31}P topical magnetic resonance. Nature 287:736–738

Holland GN, Hawkes RC, Moore WS (1980) Nuclear magnetic resonance (NMR) tomography of the brain: Coronal and sagittal sections. J Comput Assist Tomogr 4:429–433

Hoult DI, Lauterbur PC (1979) The sensitivity of the zeugmatographic experiment involving human samples. J Magn Reson 34:425–433

Kumar A, Welti D, Ernst RR (1975) NMR fourier zeugmatography. J Magn Reson 18:69–83

Lauterbur PC (1973) Image formation by induced local interactions: Examples employing nuclear magnetic resonance. Nature 242:190–191

Lauterbur PC, Ching-Ming Lai (1980) Zeugmatography by reconstruction from projections. IEEE Trans Nucl Sci NS-27:1227–1231

Mansfield P, Maudsley AA (1977) Medical imaging by NMR. Br J Radiol 50:188–194

Thomas A, Morris PG (1981) The effects of NMR exposure on living organisms. I. A microbial assay. Br J Radiol 54:615–621

Weisman ID, Bennett LH, Maxwell LR, Henson DE (1981) Cancer detection by NMR in the living animal. NMR basic principles and progress, vol 19: NMR in medicine. Springer, Berlin Heidelberg New York

Wolff S, Crooks LE, Brown P, Ricci H, Painter RB (1980) Tests for DNA and chromosomal damage induced by nuclear magnetic resonance imaging. Radiology 136:707–710

Initial Clinical Experience with NMR Imaging

R. E. Steiner and G. M. Bydder[1]

1 Introduction

In this paper we report our initial experience with a new nuclear magnetic resonance (NMR) machine installed at Hammersmith Hospital 4 months ago. We have now examined 25 volunteers and 60 patients in the initial phase of the clinical evaluation of the instrument.

From the results obtained so far there is little doubt that we are witnessing an important addition to existing imaging techniques. Anatomical detail within the brain can be seen with a clarity otherwise noted only in the dissection room and physiological effects due to blood flow and differences in oxygen tension are readily demonstrated. Furthermore, pathological effects of disease, such as plaques in multiple sclerosis, can be seen in detail observed previously only at post mortem.

The results have been made possible by the developmental work of Dr. Ian Young and his team at the Central Research Laboratories at Thorn EMI Ltd. This team began design work on an NMR machine in 1976 and 2 years later constructed an instrument based on a resistive magnet which produced head images of good quality (*Hounsfield* 1980). Following further development, a more sophisticated

1 Department of Diagnostic Radiology, Royal Postgraduate Medical School, Hammersmith Hospital, DuCane Road, GB-London W12 OHS

scanner, based on a cryomagnet, was constructed and installed at Hammersmith Hospital for clinical evaluation in 1981.

Prior to this installation Professor Doyle and his group at the Royal Post-graduate Medical School, Hammersmith Hospital, made some fundamental observations in animals and human volunteers using the original resistive magnet scanner, these observations having provided the basis for the present clinical evaluation on the new cryomagnetic scanner.

In this paper we firstly describe the new NMR machine, summarise the important observations made by Professor Doyle on the earlier instrument and finally outline some results from the clinical evaluation.

2 Machine Description

A cryogenic magnet constructed by Oxford Instruments is used to produce a magnetic field B_0 of 0.1–0.3 T with a stability of better than 1 part in 10^7 per hour. The field's uniformity is 5 parts in 10^6 over a 28 cm imaging diameter and 10 parts in 10^6 over a 55 cm diameter. The super-conducting solenoid of this magnet is placed in liquid helium at 4 °K. This is surrounded by a vacuum and an outer compartment of liquid nitrogen to reduce the helium boil-off rate, which is typically 0.31 per hour. The magnet has a clear bore of 105 cm and an access bore of 75.5 cm. Two pairs of coils placed inside the bore of the cryomagnet produce a gradient in the B_z component of the magnet field which varies linearly in the orthogonal plane. One set of coils produced a linear gradient of B_z along the X direction while another set, rotated through 90° with respect to the first set, produces a Y-varying field. By vector addition of these two fields, a radial (r) gradient is generated. The third gradient coil is a Helmholtz pair, wound anti-parallel to produce a variation in the magnetic component B_z in the Z direction. This set of coils is used for slice selection.

RF transmitter and receiver coils are placed inside the gradient coils. A circular receiver coil is used for head scanning and an elliptical coil for body scanning. Since the signal-to-noise ratio of the NMR signal is improved by tight coupling of the coil with the patient, these coils have been designed to within the dimensions of the 97th percentile of the US population.

The system is centrally controlled by a Data General S/250 Eclipse computer. Software control of the amplifiers, timing sequences and signal sampling allows a variety of scanning modes to be used. XY as well as r Θ scanning and reconstruction are available. Repeated FID rapid-repeated FID, inversion-recovery ($180°-\tau$ $-90°$) and spin-echo ($90° - \tau - 180°$) sequences are used and have been described more fully elsewhere (*Doyle* et al. 1981; *Young* et al. 1982). By appropriate choice of τ and repetition rates, images are produced with varying dependence on proton density, T_1 and T_2.

In all scanning sequences 90° RF pulses are applied, together with a slice-selecting time-varying magnetic field gradient along the Z direction. During signal recovery, the X and Y gradients are applied, forming an r gradient which alters the precessional frequency of the nuclei, and spatially encodes the reradiated RF

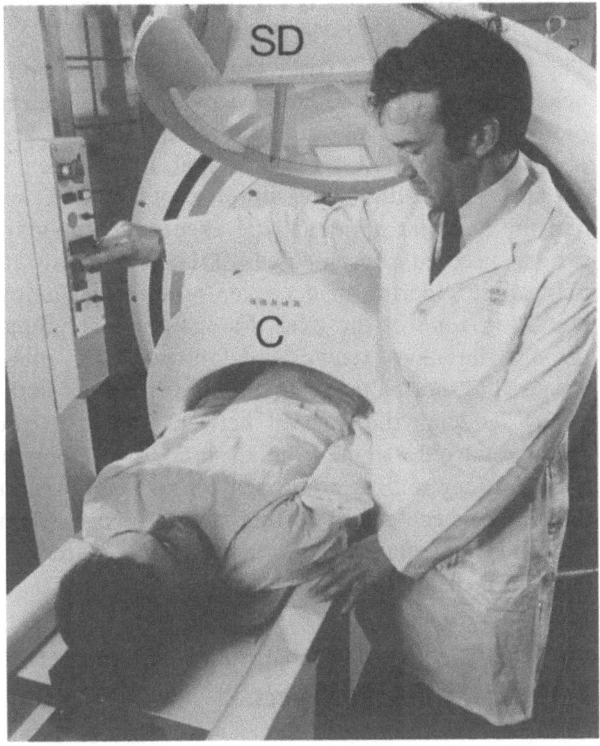

Fig. 1. General view of the NMR machine and patient handling. The patient is positioned inside the transmitter and receiver coils (*C*). The patient and coil are then slid into the magnet. The screening door (*SD*) is shown open

energy which is detected by the receiver coil. In the r Θ system, the magnitude of the r gradient is constant but the direction steps round in 1° intervals so that 180° angles are required for each image. Reconstruction is by Fourier transformation on each angle, filtered by an appropriate function, followed by back projection. In XY scanning either of the X or Y gradients is held constant while the other is stepped in magnitude. Reconstruction requires a two-dimensional Fourier transformation.

The magnitude of the X and Y gradients alters according to the size of the imaged area and hence the resolution alters between head and body scanning but is always less than 2.5 mm. The slice width can be altered by changing the RF and Z gradient field shapes, but is usually chosen at about 9 mm.

The scanner is installed in a purpose-built building. Apart from the avoidance of iron girders and large units of equipment within a few metres of the magnetic system, there are few special building requirements beyond a three-phase power supply, cooling water and computer room air conditioning.

Picture quality is degraded by interference which may be machine generated or external and screening doors are placed at the ends of the magnetic system to reduce this. Patient handling is illustrated in Fig. 1.

3 Initial Studies on the Prototype NMR Imaging System

The high level of soft tissue contrast obtained with inversion-recovery images has been emphasized by Professor Doyle. This is seen in most dramatic fashion in the brain, where striking differentiation between grey and white matter can be observed (*Doyle* et al. 1981; *Gore* et al. 1982, to be published).

The value of direct measurement of T_1 and T_2 was recognised in animal studies and the fact that paramagnetic agents such as manganese and molecular oxygen can be used to shorten tissue T_1 was demonstrated. In the rabbit intravenous manganese chloride in a concentration of 20 µmol/kg approximately halves the relaxation time of the liver. Manganese is retained by the liver and its passage through the biliary tract can be followed by T_1 imaging. Similarly, inhaled oxygen was used to shorten the relaxation time of blood in the left ventricular cavity.

By reducing the interval between pulses in proton density scans, saturation effects reduce the signal from all static tissue elements whilst blood moving into the slice between pulses continues to give a maximum signal. By decreasing the interval between pulses further slower flowing elements can be demagnetised, so that only elements which are flowing rapidly are imaged. This technique provides a basis for measurement of flow.

4 Overall Clinical Aspects

The work performed on the prototype machine provided a basis for the evaluation of the later machine and much of the clinical work has been a confirmation and extension of the earlier animal and human volunteer studies.

We are grateful for the interest and advice of the National Radiological Protection Board who have taken a lead in the study of the safety aspects of NMR and issued guidelines for clinical imaging (*NRPB* 1980). All examinations in this study have been conducted in accordance with these guidelines.

The majority of scans performed have been of the repeated FID and inversion-recovery mode taking 3 and 4.2 min respectively. Between 4 and 15 slices have been performed in each patient. Image processing which initially took 4 min now takes about 1.5 min.

On the images display system, repeated FID images which principally reflect proton density are shown with higher proton concentration at the light end of the grey scale and vice versa. Inversion-recovery images are displayed so that tissues with a short T_1 appear towards the white end of the grey scale and tissues with a long T_1 appear at the dark end. Tissues with a low proton density also appear dark.

In order to provide a comparison, virtually all patients who have had NMR scans have also had CT scans. These have been performed on a Siemens Somatom 2 whole body scanner operating at 125 kVp and 230 mAs. Ten-second scans have been obtained in the head. Five-second scans during suspended respiration have been performed in the body. Oral contrast has been used routinely for bowel labelling in the abdomen and intravenous contrast enhancement when clinically indicated.

5 The Brain

The oustanding feature of the brain images is the striking grey-white matter differentiation seen with the inversion-recovery sequence (Fig. 2). White matter can be seen from the central regions of the brain to sub-cortical level with a clarity quite unattainable with CT. The basal ganglia and thalamus are defined by the surrounding white matter and CSF. Other areas of grey matter such as the insular cortex are also easily seen (*Doyle* et al. 1981).

While the white rim around the CT image represents bone, that around the NMR image represents subcutaneous fat and yellow bone marrow. The inner and outer tables of the skull are frequently seen as parallel dark lines (since cortical bone contains little hydrogen and gives a low signal) with bone marrow between them.

Cerebral infarction is characterised by a loss of grey-white matter contrast and this change has been seen in areas where no abnormality is detectable with CT. The margins of the loss of contrast define the boundaries of the area of infarction and in cases where this change is seen on CT the correspondence with NMR is good (Fig. 3).

Tumours generally show an increased relaxation time, appearing dark on inversion-recovery images. Cerebral oedema is also associated with a prolonged relaxation time. Mass effects are seen in a very similar way to CT. Even with very obvious tumours on the inversion-recovery image very little change is usually seen in the repeated FID image apart from compression of the ventricular system.

The grey-white matter contrast seen in normal patients provides a basis for visualising abnormalities in neurological disease in which demyelination is a feature of the pathological process. In this respect multiple sclerosis (MS) has been

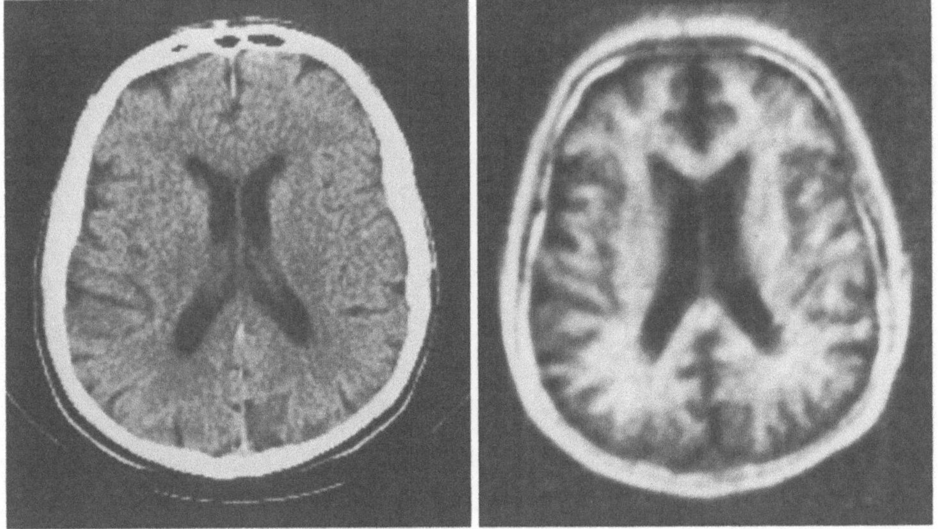
a   b

Fig. 2a, b. Normal brain: CT (**a**) and inversion-recovery (**b**) scans. The ventricular systems are seen in corresponding positions. There is considerable differentiation between grey and white matter on the NMR scan

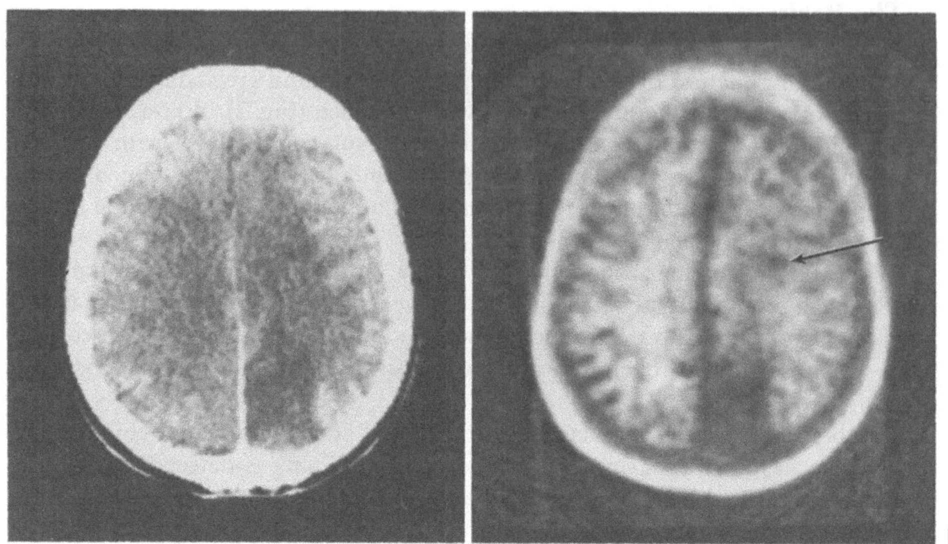

Fig. 3a, b. Cerebral infarction: CT (**a**) and inversion-recovery (**b**) scans. The region of infarction is seen within right posterior cerebral artery territory on both scans. An additional small area of infarction is probably present more anteriorly (*arrow*)

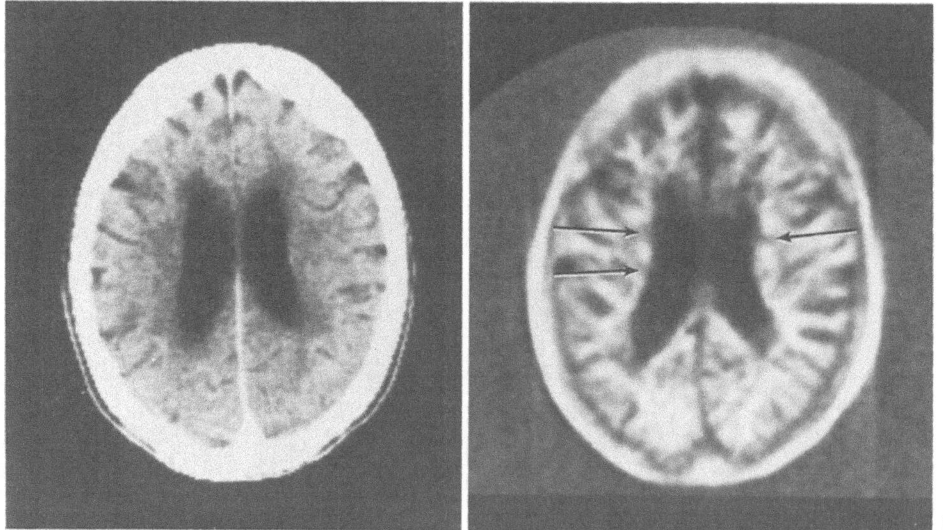

Fig. 4a, b. Multiple sclerosis: CT (**a**) and inversion-recovery (**b**) scans. Abnormal areas are noted at the anterior and posterior aspects of the lateral ventricle on both sides. In addition abnormal areas are seen at the lateral margins of the lateral ventricles on the NMR scan (*arrows*)

a disease of particular interest. While lesions can be detected with CT (*Gyldensted* 1976) it is known from CT examination of cadaver brains (*Haughton* et al. 1979) that the proportion of lesions detected is only a small fraction of the total number present. Since there may be major problems in the diagnosis of MS in the early stages, this disease provides an important potential clinical application for NMR imaging. In all ten patients so far examined lesions have been demonstrated on a scale far in excess of that seen with CT (*Young* et al. 1981). There are difficulties in distinguishing lesions from artefacts and partial volume effects from sulci and the ventricular system, nevertheless in each case where a lesion was seen on CT it was also seen on NMR and lesions were seen where no abnormality was detected with CT (Fig. 4).

NMR may prove valuable in degenerative neurological disease, as well as diseases involving demyelination, by virtue of its capacity to separate the grey and white matter components in disease.

In a general sense, CT is much more accurate in "neurosurgical" disease such as tumour, abscess, haemorrhage and hydrocephalus than it is in "neurological" disease. Since many neurological diseases involve an element of demyelination and thus may be well demonstrated with NMR, CT and NMR may prove to be complementary for imaging of the brain.

6 The Posterior Fossa

Separate consideration is given to the posterior fossa for several reasons. The lack of bone artefact with NMR gives it an advantage cover CT, and the grey-white

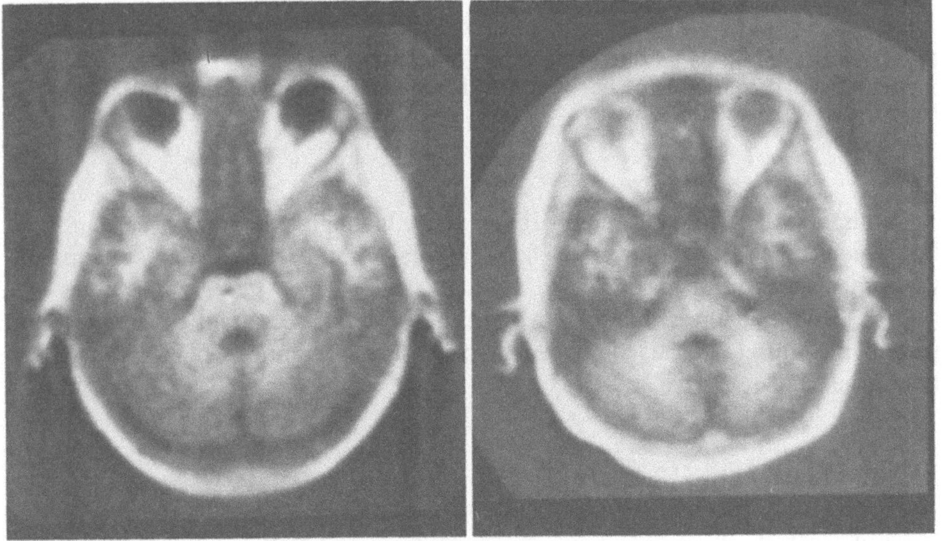

Fig. 5a, b. Normal posterior fossa: inversion-recovery scans through the upper (a) and lower (b) pons. The anterior margin of the pons is well shown (a) and the middle cerebellar peduncle is seen extending posteriorly (b)

matter differentiation available with inversion-recovery images enables internal structure to be seen within the brain-stem and cerebellum. Also, rapid-repeated FID sequences can be utilised to highlight the internal carotid, vertebral and basilar arteries as a basis for the measurement of blood flow.

Figure 5a shows the upper pons, the anterior margin of which is particularly well defined. In Fig. 5b the middle cerebellar peduncle is seen as a large white matter structure extending from the pons into the cerebellum. Posterior to the fourth ventricle the vermis of the cerebellum is seen. The middle cerebellar peduncle, although not previously visualised by any other technique, is likely to become a major anatomical landmark within the posterior fossa.

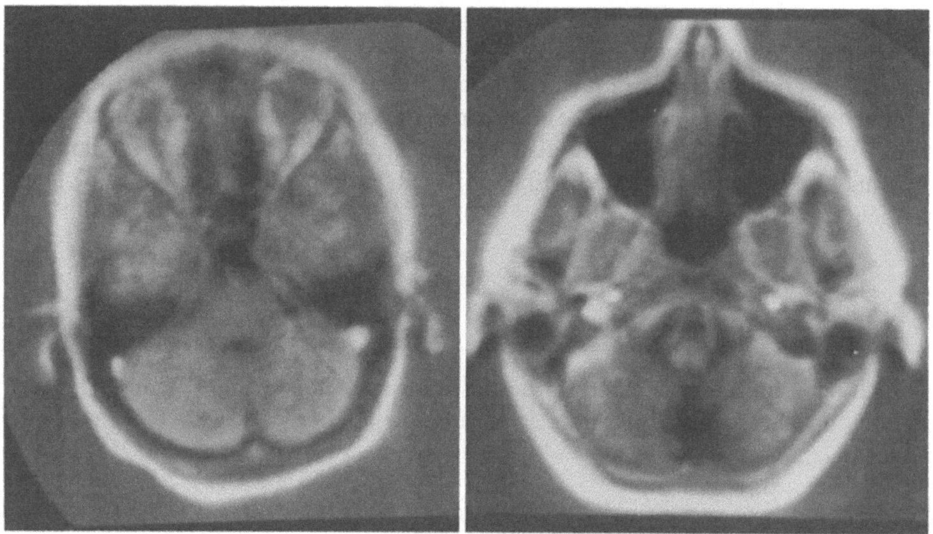

a   b

Fig. 6a, b. Normal posterior fossa: rapid repeated FID scans (**a** and **b**). The transverse sinuses are well shown (**a**) and at a lower level the internal carotid arteries, jugular veins and basilar arteries are seen (**b**)

Utilisation of a rapid-repeated FID sequence highlights the transverse sinuses in this region (Fig. 6a). At a lower level, the internal carotid arteries, jugular veins and vertebral arteries are seen (Fig. 6b).

It is likely that the scope for NMR in the posterior fossa will be greater than that in the supratentorial compartment because of limitations of CT caused by bone artefact (*Young* et al. 1981).

7 The Heart

Scans through the heart are shown in Fig. 7. Repeated FID images which largely reflect proton density show little contrast between blood and myocardium, but these structures are clearly distinguished using the inversion-recovery sequence. In

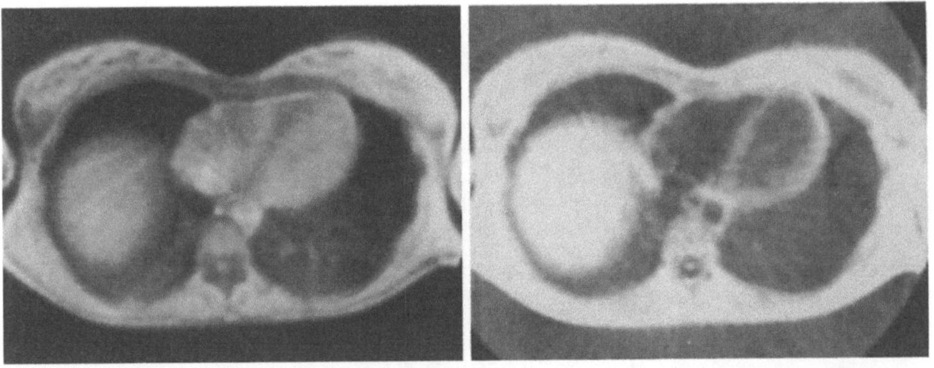

a   b

Fig. 7a, b. Normal heart: repeated FID (**a**) and inversion-recovery (**b**) scans. The septum is barely seen on the repeated FID scan (**a**) but the cardiac chambers, septum and free wall of the left ventricle are seen on the inversion-recovery scan (**b**)

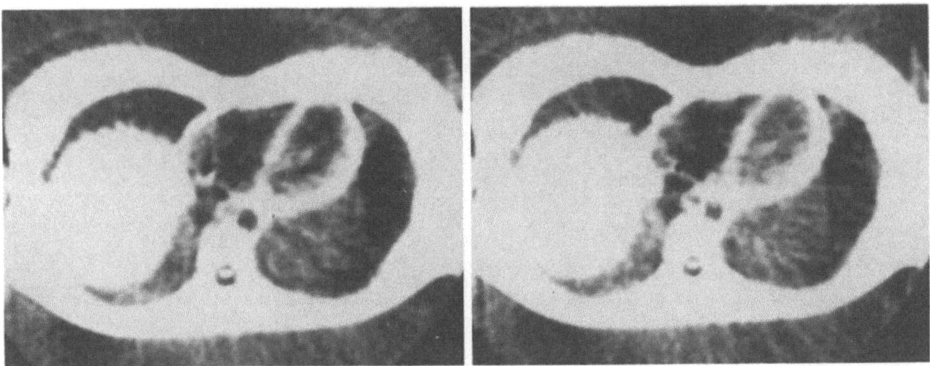

a   b

Fig. 8a, b. Normal heart: inversion-recovery scans breathing air (**a**) and 100% oxygen (**b**). The narrowly windowed scans show changes within the left ventricular cavity and an apparent thickening of the free wall of the left ventricle following 100% oxygen

six volunteers differences have been seen in the spin-lattice relaxation time (T_1) of blood in the left and right ventricular cavities. On breathing 100% oxygen this effect is increased (Fig. 8). Although the effect is small and further work will be required to correlate arterial blood tensions directly with relaxation time, the paramagnetic properties of oxygen may provide the basis for a new approach to imaging metabolic processes.

8 The Liver

In spite of respiratory movement during the 4.2-min scan time causing blurring, the high level of soft tissue contrast on inversion-recovery images enables the liver to

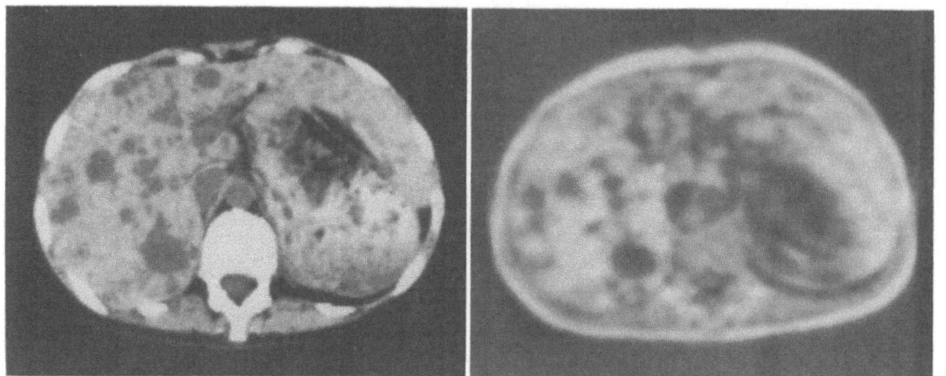

Fig. 9a, b. Liver metastases: CT (**a**) and inversion-recovery scans (**b**). Although the inversion-recovery scan appears blurred due to respiratory motion the multiple metastases are readily seen

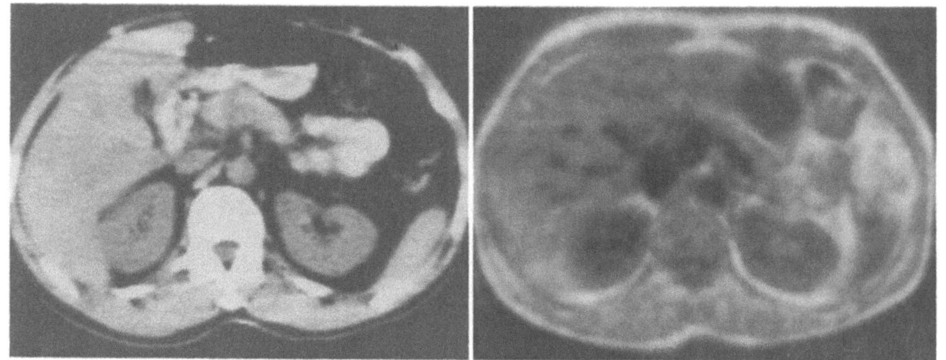

Fig. 10a, b. Cirrhosis: CT (**a**) and inversion-recovery (**b**) scans. On the inversion-recovery scan the liver parenchyma appears unusually dark due to its prolonged spin-lattice relaxation time

be seen with considerable clarity. Intrahepatic blood vessels and bile ducts appear dark against the grey of normal liver parenchyma.

From our initial experience with 32 patients (*Doyle* et al. 1982) focal disease is easily seen with both CT and NMR, although the diagnosis of hepatic infarct was only correctly recognised with NMR in one case and an area of focal atrophy was only seen with NMR in another case. Metastases are easily seen with both techniques (Fig. 9).

In diffuse disease the pattern is more varied. In steatosis CT is virtually diagnostic while NMR is unhelpful. In many other conditions information of varying specificity is contributed by both techniques, but in two cases of cirrhosis and one case of primary biliary cirrhosis NMR alone showed an abnormality.

Cirrhosis is of particular interest (Fig. 10). In addition to the morphological abnormalities which are seen in a similar way to CT, T_1 is prolonged to varying degrees. Exceptions to this pattern may be found in forms of cirrhosis in which excessive copper (which is paramagnetic) is accumulated, such as primary biliary cirrhosis and Wilson's disease.

Overall, in liver disease T_1 values are a sensitive but relatively non-specific diagnostic parameter, being shortened in diseases where there is excessive copper or iron (which is also paramagnetic) and lengthened in a variety of conditions including hepatitis, cirrhosis, infarction and tumours.

In an important study of 30 patients *Smith* et al. (1981) compared NMR favourably with isotope scanning and ultrasonography and drew attention to the value of T_1 in liver diagnosis. This represented the first comparative study of NMR and our results support their findings.

9 The Pancreas

The pancreas has a relaxation time similar to that of liver, and disease processes such as tumour and pancreatitis have the effect of lengthening this (*Young* et al. 1982). As a result of these diseases the pancreas may be difficult to visualise because its relaxation time becomes similar to that of adjacent fluid-filled loops of bowel. We have used diluted oral ferric chloride solution in volunteers and shown that it can be used as a bowel labelling agent (*Young* et al., to be published a) but more work will be required in order to ascertain whether or not NMR has a useful role in distinguishing diffuse and focal disease within the pancreas.

10 The Adrenals

High resolution images can be obtained by increasing the gradient fields and these are particularly useful in imaging small structures such as the adrenal gland. The images tend to be noisy but better quality is usually obtained by increasing the scan time from 4.2 to 8.4 min (*Young* et al. 1982).

11 Kidneys

The most striking feature about the kidney images is the differentiation of cortex and medulla utilising the inversion-recovery sequence. The columns of Berthin are also seen extending centrally. Perirenal fat is clearly seen around the kidney. In a patient with renal failure due to chronic glomerulonephritis the NMR scan displayed both shrunken kidneys and loss of the cortical margin, whereas a well-defined cortical rim was seen on the patient's transplanted kidney. If NMR is to have a specific role in renal disease it appears likely to be in diffuse parenchymal disease, rather than focal diseases which are already well demonstrated with existing techniques (*Young* et al. 1982).

12 The Spinal Cord

The high resolution mode of the scanner is useful for visualising the spinal cord.
Grey and white matter are seen within the cord and CSF appears as a dark area,
with white epidural fat beyond this. Nerve roots within the cauda equina have also
been identified.

13 Other Regions

A purpose-designed neck coil is presently being commissioned and detail of the
cervical spinal cord is evident. Scans of the limbs are of interest. The cortex of long
bones appears black with central white-yellow marrow, in direct contrast to CT
where the cortex appears white and the yellow marrow black. Soft dissue detail in
muscle is well displayed.

14 Conclusions

Although the clinical evaluation has only been in progress for 4 months an im-
pressive series of images is already available as a guide to the future role of NMR
in clinical practice.

Within the brain grey and white matter have been differentiated to a remarkable degree and the absence of bone artefact has opened up new possibilities for
imaging the posterior fossa.

The heart is readily visualised and effects of oxygen on blood relaxation time
have been observed.

A variety of diseases of the liver have been recognised, and the kidney appears
particularly promising because of the differentiation between cortex and medulla
observed in normal subjects.

High resolution scans are useful for visualising the adrenal and spinal cord.

Our first few months of clinical work with out present machine have been a
period of great interest, and there is now little doubt that NMR will make a major
contribution to diagnostic imaging in the near future.

Acknowledgements. The considerable help and encouragement given by the
Department of Health and Social Security is gratefully acknowledged. The
particular contribution of Mr. *Gordon Higson* and Mr. *John Williams* is especially
worthy of mention.

References

Doyle FH, Gore JC, Pennock JM, Bydder GM, Orr JS, Steiner RE, Young IR, Burl M, Clow
    H, Gilderdale DJ, Bailes DR, Walters PE (1981a) Imaging of the brain by nuclear mag-
    netic resonance. Lancet II:53–57

Doyle FH, Gore JC, Pennock JM (1981 b) Relaxation rate enhancement observed in vivo by NMR imaging. J Comp Assist Tomogr 5:295–296

Doyle FH, Pennock JM, Banks LM, McDonnell MJ, Bydder GM, Steiner RE, Young IR, Clarke GJ, Pasmore T, Gilderdale DJ (1982) Nuclear magnetic resonance (NMR) imaging of the liver: Initial Experience. AJR 193–200

Gore JC, Doyle FH, Pennock JM (1981) Nuclear magnetic resonance (NMR) imaging at Hammersmith Hospital. SPIE 273:8–10

Gore JC, Doyle FH, Pennock JM (to be published) Relaxation rate enhancement observed in vivo by NMR imaging. In: James AE, Partain CL (eds) NMR Imaging Saunders, Philadelphia

Gyldensted C (1976) Computer tomography of the brain in multiple sclerosis. Acta Neurol Scand 53:386–389

Haughton VM, Khang-cheng Ho, Williams AL, Elderick OP (1979) CT detection of demyalinating plaques in multiple sclerosis. AJR 132:213–215

Hounsfield GN (1980) Computed medical imaging. J Comput Assist Tomogr 4:665–674

NRPB (1980) Exposure to nuclear magnetic resonance clinical imaging 1980. Available from the Secretary, NRPB, Harwell, Oxon OX 11 ORQ, UK

Smith FW, Mallard JR, Reid A, Hutchinson JMS (1981) Nuclear magnetic resonance imaging in liver disease. Lancet I:963–966

Young IR, Clarke GJ, Bailes DR, Pennock JM, Doyle FH, Bydder GM (to be published a) The use of paramagnetic contrast agents in nuclear magnetic resonance (NMR) imaging

Young IR, Burl M, Clarke GJ, Hall AS, Pasmore T, Collins AJ, Smith DT, Orr JS, Bydder GM, Doyle FH, Greenspan RH, Steiner RE (1981) Posterior fossa: magnetic resonance imaging properties. AJR 137: 895–901

Young IR, Bailes DR, Burl M, Collins AG, Smith DT, McDonnell MJ, Banks LM, Bydder GM, Steiner RE (1982) Initial clinical evaluation of a whole body NMR scanner. J Comp Assist Tomogr 6: 1–18

Young IR, Hall AS, Pallis CA, Legg NJ, Bydder GM, Steiner RE (1981) Nuclear magnetic resonance imaging of the brain in multiple sclerosis. Lancet 138: 1063–1066

NMR Imaging of the Liver and Kidney

F. W. Smith [1]

1 Introduction

Over the past 2–3 years major advances in nuclear magnetic resonance (NMR) imaging have been made. This new non-invasive imaging technique has been developed to the extent that images of the human body can be made which are comparable in appearance to early X-ray CT scans (*Moore* et al. 1980; *Doyle* et al. 1981; *Smith* 1981). The images may be displayed as axial sections in a similar way to X-ray CT, but here the similarity ends. NMR images are composed of either different proton density or proton spin-lattice relaxation time (T_1) measurements of the water in different body tissues, whereas X-ray CT images are composed of different X-ray coefficients of absorption. By studying the different proton compositions of different tissues it is possible to produce anatomically accurate images of the human body and to differentiate the different tissues therein. The normal grey and white matter of the brain have been clearly demonstrated (*Moore* et al. 1980) as have intracerebral tumours (*Doyle* et al. 1981) and other intracranial pathology (*Smith* to be published). In the abdomen it is possible to demonstrate the liver, spleen, kidneys and large blood vessels on the T_1 images and to demonstrate the vertebral bodies and pelvic bones using the proton density images. A preliminary study of the liver, comparing NMR with both ultrasound and radionuclide liver scan, has shown that NMR is at least as sensitive as either of them in demonstrating liver tumours and hepatocellular disease, and is more specific than either of them in differentiating benign from malignant tumours

1 Aberdeen Royal Infirmary, Foresterhill, GB-Aberdeen AB9 2ZB

(*Smith* et al. 1981 a, b, c). Similarly NMR imaging has been shown to be an accurate method of diagnosing the nature of renal masses (*Smith* et al. 1981 d).

The "Spin warp" method of NMR imaging is used in Aberdeen and all the images used in this paper were produced by this technique. The technique has been developed by a team of physicists led by Dr. James Hutchison and is well described elsewhere (*Hutchinson* et al. 1980; *Edelstein* et al. 1980; *Mallard* et al. 1980).

2 Imaging Technique

The NMR imaging technique is based on measuring the response of the hydrogen protons within tissues mostly water and fat to an applied radio-frequency radiation. The Aberdeen imager is based on a four-coil, air-cored magnet which produces a magnetic field of 0.04 Tesla and a consequent NMR frequency of 1.7 MHz for the hydrogen protons of body tissues.

The imager produces two types of image. The first uses proton density as the imaging parameter, and the second uses the proton spin-lattice relaxation time or T_1. When a patient is placed in a strong electromagnetic field, a proportion of the protons align with the magnetic field and precess around it at a definite resonant frequency. If a radio-frequency pulse of the same frequency is beamed into the patient, the protons absorb energy and change their alignment relative to the applied magnetic field. When a 90° radio-frequency pulse is used, this sets them precessing at 90° to the field. When the irradiating pulse is ended, the protons, one by one relax back to their original alignment and re-radiate the absorbed energy. This re-radiated resonant frequency is detected and measured, the size of the signal being related to the number of protons involved and is known as the PROTON DENSITY. After a 180° radio-frequency pulse, the proton spins are completely inverted, and the length of time required for their relaxation is associated with their environment. The intensity of the emitted radiation falls exponentially at a rate characteristic of its environment or lattice of which it is a part, a measurement known as PROTON SPIN-LATTICE RELAXATION TIME or T_1. T_1 depends essentially on the relative proportions of free and protein-bound water within the tissues under examination. The easier it is for the protons to pass energy to neighbouring protons, the more rapidly they will relax to their original state and the faster is the fall in the intensity of the re-radiated signal. Thus, tissues with a large amount of bound water, such as muscle and liver, have a short T_1, whilst fluids such as urine and ascitic fluid have long values. Furthermore it has been shown in in vitro experiments that malignant tissues have longer relaxation times than the equivalent normal tissues (*Damadian* et al. 1973), an observation which has been substantiated by our early in vivo work in Aberdeen (*Smith* et al. 1981 b, d).

The data for each section, which includes both proton density and T_1 information, are collected from 128, 1-s pulse sequences, Fourier transformed into two 64×64 element arrays which are then interpolated to 256×256 arrays and displayed on a visual display unit in either monochrome or colour using 16 coded colour levels. Each pair of sections (PD and T_1) take just over 2 min to collect. Recently a technique for collecting 256 pulse sequences, which are then trans-

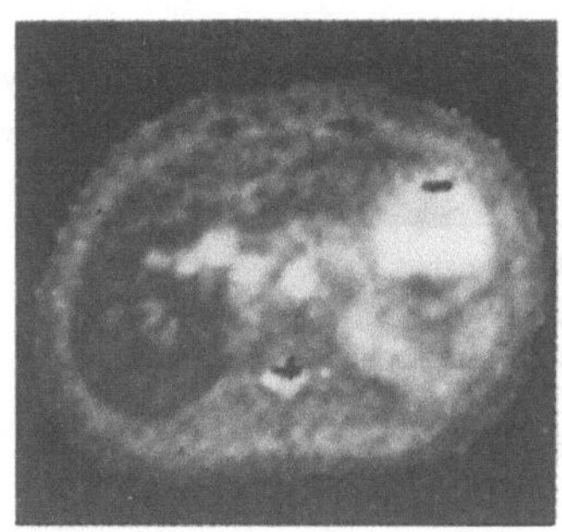

Fig. 1. All sections are viewed on the acepted CT format so that the patient's left is on the reader's right. 128×128 NMR image through the upper abdomen demonstrating the normal liver which appears black with white portal tracts and is just visible. The spleen and upper pole of the left kidney are seen as grey, with the stomach lying anterior to them, white with a small black air bubble. The aorta is clearly seen anterior to the vertebral body, which is not clearly demonstrated on this T_1 image

Table 1. Proton spin-lattice relaxation times for normal tissues measured using a 1.7 MHz pulsed radio frequency

Tissue	Relaxation time (T_1) milliseconds
Liver	140 – 170
Spleen	250 – 290
Pancreas	180 – 200
Bile	250 – 300
Blood	340 – 370
Kidney	300 – 340
Bladder	180 – 220
Prostate	250 – 325
Urine	800 – 1000
Ascitic fluid	500 – 1000

formed to 128×128 element arrays before being interpolated to 256×256 and displayed, has been developed. The collection time is just over 4 min but the image quality is four times better than the earlier 64×64 images. Thus, data may be collected in just over either 2 or 4 min, which compares favourably with other NMR imaging systems and early CT scanners.

3 Tissue Characterisation

Of the two available proton measurements, proton density and T_1, it is the T_1 measurements which are proving to be the more useful for soft tissue characterisation. The proton density images give a display of proton concentration which does not vary significantly from soft tissue to soft tissue. There are however significant differences between bone and soft tissue and between fluid-filled organs and soft tissue when viewed on the proton density images. These images are therefore very useful when studying bone or fluid-filled structures such as the urinary bladder. On our system both bone and fluid show as black whilst the soft tissues show as shades of grey.

Soft tissue organs on the other hand are best demonstrated and studied on the T_1 images (Fig. 1). Individual soft tissues have their own characteristic protein/

Table 2. Proton spin-lattice relaxation times for some pathological conditions measured using a 1.7 MHz pulsed radio frequency

Tissue	Relaxation time (T_1) milliseconds
Cirrhosis	180 – 300
Hepatoma	300 – 450
Cholangiocarcinoma	300 – 450
Metastases	300 – 450
Haemangioma	340 – 370
Simple cyst	800 – 1000
Pancreatitis	200 – 275
Carcinoma pancreas	275 – 400
Carcinoma kidney	400 – 450
Metastases kidney	400 – 450
Simple cyst	600 – 1000
Abscess	390 – 420
Acute tubular necrosis	400 – 420
Carcinoma bladder	300 – 350
Carcinoma prostate	350 – 450

water composition, which displays as characteristic T_1 values in the images (Table 1). In the abdomen differentiation of the liver, spleen and kidneys is simple, as is the demonstration of the major blood vessels, inflammatory disease of the liver and kidneys and the differentiation of benign from malignant tumours. In general terms malignant tissue appears to have a T_1 which is about 25% longer than its equivalent normal tissue (Table 2).

4 Contraindications

During the past year over 250 patients and 40 volunteers have been imaged in Aberdeen, having exposures to a 0.04 Tesla electromagnetic field and 1.7 MHz pulsed radio-frequency, for periods ranging from 4–30 min. No evidence of any objective or subjective, short- or medium-term ill effect arising from this technique has been observed.

Epilepsy was formerly considered to be a contraindication to NMR imaging. Experience with four epileptic patients and one volunteer who suffers from epilepsy suggests that no ill effect is experienced by these suffers and we no longer consider epilepsy to be a contraindication to NMR imaging.

Similarly, recent myocardial infarction was considered to be a contraindication. Whilst we have not imaged any patient who has had a myocardial infarct in the 14 days prior to imaging, we have examined three patients in their 3rd week after infarction with no disturbance to cardiac rhythm, suggesting that it is probably more safe than previously thought.

Patients who have cardiac pacemakers in situ are not imaged because the pulsed radiofrequency gradients and static magnetic field will both disrupt the

Table 3

Organ	Patient numbers
Liver	76
Pancreas	15
Kidneys	26
Prostate	17
Renal transplant	15
Total	149

electronic control of the pacemaker and interfere with electrical conduction in the leads, resulting in pacemaker failure.

Because it is almost impossible to prove categorically that any new system is totally safe, it being easier to demonstrate hazards, it is prudent not to investigate pregnant patients until sufficient small animal work has been completed to show that there is no teratogenic effect associated with NMR frequencies in the range to be used for diagnostic purposes. Therefore, all pregnant patients are excluded at present and the radiological 10-day rule is applied to all females of child-bearing age.

The presence of large metallic joint prostheses causes no discomfort to the patient during imaging, but does cause a large artifact on the image. A large irregular area of no signal is seen around the metallic object, which, if close to the area of interest, will cause problems in interpretation.

NMR imaging is considered to be a safe, totally non-invasive technique for producing tomographic sections similar in appearance to X-ray CT, but without the use and small hazard of X-rays.

5 Clinical Application

Of the 250 patients studied so far 149 have had disease of either liver, pancreas or the urinary tract (Table 3). In an effort to evaluate the sensitivity and specificity of the NMR imaging technique, all the patients studied have been fully diagnosed by other conventional means, including biopsy wherever possible. As far as possible the NMR images have been compared with abdominal ultrasound and nuclear medicine liver scan in the cases of liver disease and intravenous urography in the cases of renal disease. Unfortunately no whole-body X-ray CT scanner is available at present to compare with the NMR images.

5.1 Liver

Normal liver tissue has a T_1 value in the range 140–170 ms making it easily recognisable, surrounded by the abdominal wall, bowel and overlying lung (Fig. 2).

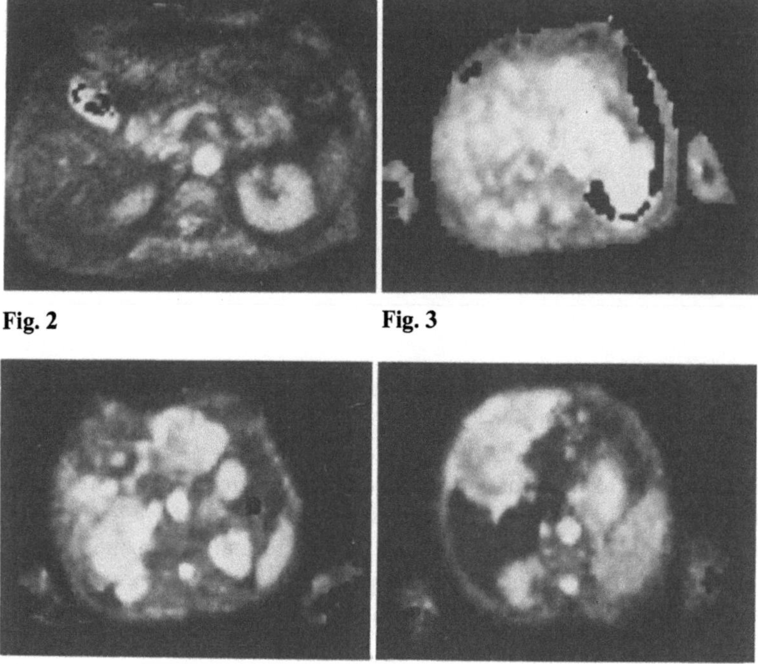

Fig. 2   **Fig. 3**

Fig. 4   **Fig. 5**

Fig. 2. 128×128 T_1 section through the liver showing the normal gall bladder and common bile duct. The upper pole of the right kidney is just visible, as is the left kidney

Fig. 3. 64×64, T_1 image of a liver containing multiple small metastases (white) throughout the liver, from a primary carcinoma of the oesophagus. The base of the left lung is seen as black

Fig. 4. 64×64, T_1 image of the liver showing multiple large metastases from a primary carcinoma of the rectum

Fig. 5. 64×64, T_1 image demonstrating a large cholangiocarcinoma in a liver involved with haemochromatosis. The tumour appears white and the liver black. Note the large white spleen

The normal spleen, because of its vascularity, has a T_1 in the range 250–290 ms, which has been noted to be lower in cases of haemolytic anaemia. Blood in the major blood vessels has a value of between 340–370 ms. The portal tracts are occasionally seen within the liver as is the gall bladder when present.

When the liver becomes inflamed due to active hepatitis, there is a generalised increase in T_1 in the range 180–300 ms. This same elevation of T_1 is seen in cirrhosis, where in the early stages of the disease the increased relaxation time, which is seen as a whiter shade of grey, is confined to around the portal tracts within the liver, spreading out to involve the whole liver as the disease progresses. This distinctive pattern makes the differentiation of hepatocellular disease from hepatic metastases easier than is possible with either ultrasound or sulphur colloid liver scan (*Smith* et al. 1981 b). Even when the metastases are as small as 1–2cm in diameter they are easily demonstrated by their shape, distribution and T_1 (Figs. 3, 4). The T_1 of metastases, hepatoma and cholangio-carcinoma lie in the same range (300–450 ms) and whilst there is a little overlap at around 300 ms with hepatocellular disease, the space-occupying nature of the tumours is usually evident (Fig. 5). When the center of a tumour becomes necrotic, the T_1 is further elongated (450–600 ms), making differentiation from cystic lesions theoretically difficult. Simple cystic lesions of the liver, filled with serous fluid, have a T_1 of between 800–1000 ms, whilst blood-filled cysts and haemangiomata have T_1 values similar to blood (340–370). Both these cystic lesions have thin walls and may have fibrous septae running through them, enabling easy differentiation from necrotic tumours which tend to have thicker walls. NMR will give a definite diagnosis as to the nature of the space-occupying lesion, whereas ultrasound will only tell if the lesion is cystic or solid and liver scan will simply indicate the presence of a space-occupying lesion. X-ray CT has also proved to be less accurate at demonstrating the presence of solid tumours of liver, but it remains to be seen whether or not NMR will prove to be superior to it or not. Pus has a T_1 in the range 400–450 ms, which unfortunately overlaps the tumour range and great care must be taken when differentiating between the two. However, in the search for subphrenic or subhepatic abscess, NMR is proving to be both sensitive and specific.

Ascitic fluid, because of its long T_1, is clearly seen. Its T_1 has quite a large range depending on the protein content of the fluid. In cases of cirrhosis it may be as long as between 800–1000 ms, but when a high protein is present it may be as short as 500 ms, e.g. in the Budd-Chiari syndrome. However, it is seldom as low as 400 ms and is not usually confused with intra-peritoneal pus.

5.2 Biliary Tract

The enlarged gall bladder and dilated bile ducts are clearly demonstrated on NMR images, but as yet no calculus has been demonstrated as the cause of the obstruction (Fig. 2). When the gall bladder is inflamed, as in cholecystitis, the bile within the gall bladder tends to have a longer than normal T_1. The normal T_1 which ranges from 300–500 ms may be as long as 1000 ms in some cases. It may also be as long as this when a very large volume is present in a normally large gall bladder. Differentiation from cholecystis however, is facilitated by the presence of an irregular rim of edema around the inflamed gall bladder, which has a T_1 longer than the surrounding hepatic tissue. In empyema of the gall bladder there is a further lengthening of T_1 associated with a markedly enlarged gall bladder, a fact that has been used successfully to diagnose empyema of the gall bladder in a patient following aorto-iliac surgery (*Pollet* et al. 1981).

Obstruction of the common bile duct by disease of the pancreas is demonstrated well, principally because the normal pancreas has a T_1 which is the same as the surrounding duodenum, an overlying bowel, and is not normally visualised. When inflamed, the pancreas appears as a uniformly elevated T_1 (200–275 ms) and if carcinoma is present the value is longer still (275–400 ms). In most cases of carcinoma the mass effect of the tumour is also evident. In 11 cases of unexplained upper abdominal pain we have demonstrated seven pancreatic carcinomas which had previously not been diagnosed by other means. In the other four cases no cause for the pain has even been established.

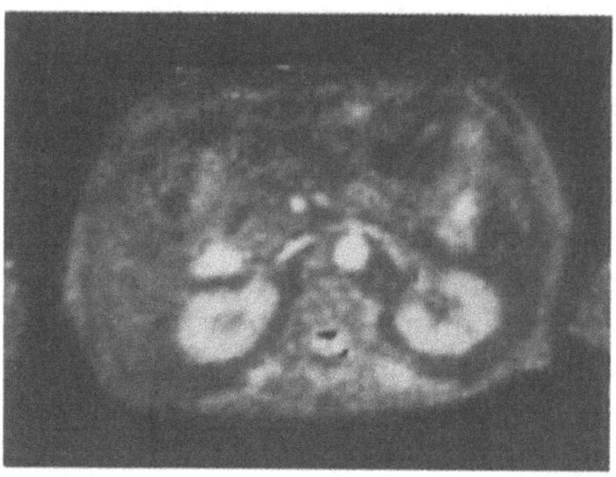
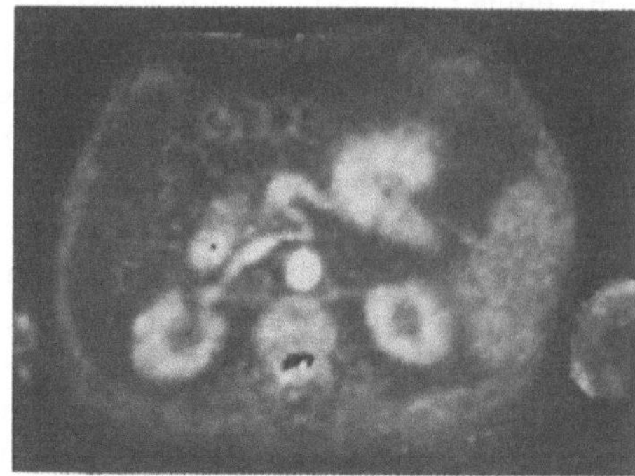

Fig. 6   **Fig. 7**

Fig. 6. 128×128 T_1 NMR image through normal kidneys, demonstrating the renal arteries as they leave the aorta. Whilst the vertebral body is not clearly outlined, the spinal canal containing CSF is clearly demarcated

Fig. 7. 128×128, T_1 images of the kidneys demonstrating the right renal artery, the superior mesenteric artery and a small cyst on the lateral aspect of the right kidney. The spleen is noted to be enlarged, as is the liver, in this patient with haemolytic anaemia

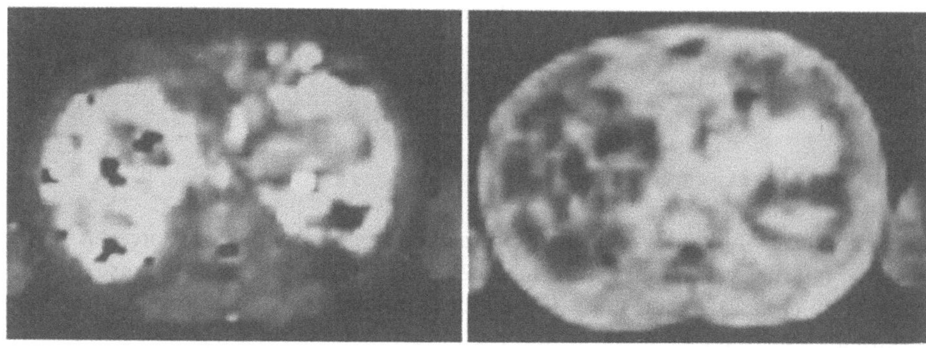

Fig. 8a. 64×64, T_1 image of large end stage polycystic kidneys. The cysts appearing as large, white, fluid-filled areas of long T_1 (800–1000). **b** Proton density image of the same polycystic kidneys as in **a**. The fluid filled cysts are more clearly demonstrated, as is the vertebral body and spinal canal

5.3 Urinary Tract

NMR T_1 images of the kidneys are very similar in appearance to X-ray CT images. In health they have a T_1 in the narrow range 300–340 ms, which does not appear to vary very much in chronic pyelonephritis or chronic glomerulonephritis. The renal parenchyma appears as a "horseshoe"-shaped organ which in the normal non-obstructed kidney has an empty renal pelvis. In most cases the renal arteries can be identified running from the aorta to the kidneys (Fig. 6). When a kidney is hydro-nephrotic, the renal pelvis and ureter may be seen to be filled with urine, which appears white on the image and has a T_1 of 800–1000 ms.

In acute tubular necrosis the renal parenchyma becomes swollen and edematous, having a T_1 in the range 400–420 ms. The collecting system is not seen due to the lack of urine formation and the fact that the swollen parenchyma has compressed it. Thus, it is a simple matter to differentiate renal from post-renal, renal failure without the use of iodinated contrast media, in a short space of time. There is no lengthy delay, waiting for the late films of an intravenous urogram to demonstrate the cause of the renal failure. Furthermore, if the cause of the renal failure is obstruction, the further axial sections can be made lower down to assess the level and nature of the obstruction.

Space-occupying lesions of the kidney are in most cases easily divided into benign cystic with a long T_1 (600–1000 ms), due to the presence of fluid within them (Figs. 7, 8) and solid tumours (400–500 ms). Some difficulty may be experienced when the centre of a tumour has become necrotic and liquified. The T_1 in these cases may be longer than 500 ms and because very often the wall of these renal tumours is thin unlike the majority of liver tumours, differentiation from a simple cyst may prove difficult. Pus has a T_1 which unfortunately overlaps with that of renal carcinomata and again care must be taken when diagnosing renal abscess. Polycystic kidneys have a characteristic appearance not unlike the CT appearances, but have the added advantage that any haemorrhagic cyst will have a shorter T_1 than a serous cyst, due to the presence of blood proteins.

Tumours of the urinary bladder are well demonstrated, especially when the bladder contains a little urine to delineate the tumour mass, which usually has a T_1 of between 300–350 ms.

Carcinoma of the prostate cannot be diagnosed by X-ray CT prior to its infiltrating through the prostatic capsule or metastasizing to the local lymph nodes. A preliminary study of 17 patients with enlarged prostate glands suggests that it is possible to diagnose carcinoma of the prostate and to differentiate it from benign prostatic hypertrophy prior to trans-urethral resection and histological examination, due to the differences in T_1 between the two conditions (Table 1).

5.4 Renal Transplants

Fifteen patients have been examined following renal allograft transplantation. Those with well-functioning, non-rejecting grafts, show a T_1 of between 325–365 ms, which is only slightly higher than that for normally situated kidneys. As allograft rejection becomes worse so the T_1 lengthens in the range 390–470 ms, which unfortunately is in the same range as kidneys with acute tubular necrosis (400–420 ms). Whilst NMR imaging may not be useful in the immediate post-operative period for the differentiation of acute tubular necrosis from rejection, it may prove useful in the assessment of renal allografts after the danger of acute tubular necrosis has passed.

6 Conclusion

This new, non-invasive, non-ionising technique for demonstrating the body organs appears, after only a very short clinical experience, to have a large potential in soft tissue diagnosis and tissue characterisation. It appears that it may fill a number of the existing gaps in the diagnostic armamentarium and complement X-ray CT, ultrasound and nuclear medicine in the investigation of the liver, pancreas, spleen and uarinary tract. A much larger series of patients with a larger variety of conditions must be examined before its true clinical role is found. With the continuing development of the NMR imaging technique it will not be long before it finds a place in regular diagnostic practice.

References

Damadian R, Zaner K, Hor D, Dimaio T, Minkoff L, Goldsmith M (1973) Nuclear magnetic resonance as a new tool in cancer research: Tumours of NMR. Ann NY Acad Sci 222:1048

Doyle FH, Gore JC, Pennock JM, Bydder GM, Orr JS, Steiner RE, Young IR, Burl M, Clow H, Gilderdale DJ, Bailles DR, Walters PE (1981) Imaging of the brain by nuclear magnetic resonance. Lancet II:53–57

Edelstein WA, Hutchison JMS, Johnson G, Redpath TW (1980) Spin warp NMR imaging and applications to human whole-body imaging. Phys Med Biol 25:751–756

Hutchison JMS, Edelstein WA, Johnson G (1980) A whole-body NMR imaging machine. J Phys E Sci Instrum 13:947–955

Mallard JR, Hutchison JMS, Edelstein WA, Ling CR, Foster MA, Johnson G (1980) In vivo NMR imaging in medicine: the Aberdeen approach, both physical and biological. Philos Trans R Soc Ser B 289:519–553

Moore WS, Holland GN, Kreel L (1980) The NMR CAT scanner – A new look at the brain. CT 4:1–7

Pollet JE, Smith FW, Mallard JR, Ah-See AK, Reid A (1981) Whole-body nuclear magnetic resonance imaging: the first report of its use in surgical practice. Br J Surg 68:493–494

Smith FW (1981) Whole-body nuclear magnetic resonance tomographic imaging. Radiography XLVII, 564: 297–300

Smith FW (to be published) Nuclear magnetic resonance imaging as applied to neuro-radiology. In: Newton TH, Potts DG (eds) Computed Tomography of the head and spine. Clavadel, New York

Smith FW, Mallard JR, Hutchison JMS, Reid A, Johnson G, Redpath TW, Selbie RD (1981 a) Clinical application of nuclear magnetic resonance. Lancet I:78–79

Smith FW, Mallard JR, Reid A, Hutchison JMS (1981 b) Nuclear magnetic resonance tomographic imaging in liver disease. Lancet I:963–966

Smith FW, Hutchison JMS, Mallard JR, Johnson G, Redpath TW, Selbie RD, Reid A, Smith CC (1981 c) Oesophageal carcinoma demonstrated by whole-body nuclear magnetic resonance imaging. Br Med J 282:510–512

Smith FW, Hutchison JMS, Mallard JR, Reid A, Johnson G, Redpath TW, Selbie RD (1981 d) Renal cyst or tumour? Differentiation by whole-body nuclear magnetic resonance imaging. Diagn Imaging 50:61–65

Digital Fluorography

P. Marhoff and M. Pfeiler[1]

1 Introduction

The term 'digital radiography' comprises three fundamentally different procedures (Figs. 1, 2) (1): The digital image of computerized tomography (CT) was the first digital X-ray image to be established in diagnostic radiology. (2) In scan projection radiography a digital X-ray image is constructed line by line, using the digital measuring system of a CT installation. (3) In digital fluoroscopy and fluorography the image itself is produced in a conventional manner and then digitalized (*Brennecke* et al. 1976; *Frost* et al. 1977; *Mistretta* et al. 1978, 1981). The question arises whether digital processing offers a substantial advantage compared with the radiological procedure of image subtraction (*Ziedses des Plantes* 1935), electronic subtraction of radiography or fluoroscopic images (pathfinder technique) (Fig. 3).

Contrary to the analog technique, digital electronics permit absolutely precise and reproducible computer operations (Fig. 4). Reproducibility does not only refer to the processing as applied to the original signals and intermediate results, but also to the playback fidelity of the temporary storage, which is indispensable for the subtraction of images depicting different temporal phases. Playback fidelity relates not so much to geometrical distortion, a problem which can never be fully resolved, e.g. in the electronic subtraction of two images produced by a TV camera, as to the noise inherent in every analog system, i.e. the additional noise imparted to a signal which has been stored and played back. Manifold storing procedures undergone by one and the same signal, in the analog method, thus lead to an increased deterioration which is due to electronic noise. This may be demonstrated when using the classic analog storage medium of radiological TV technique (Fig. 5): In converting the signal into a frequency-modulated intermediate signal, for high

---

1 Siemens AG, Medizinische Technik, Postfach 3260, D-8520 Erlangen

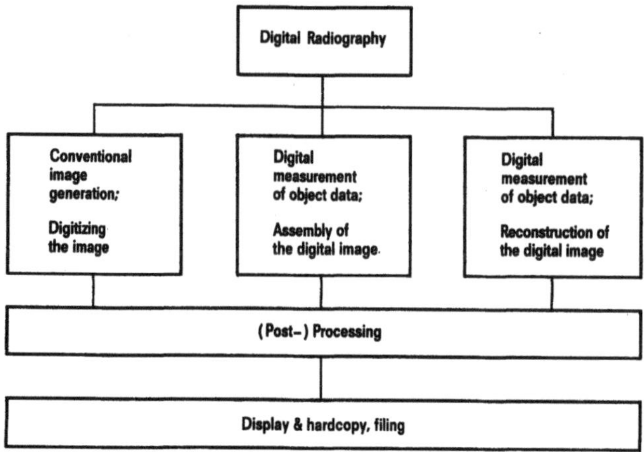

Fig. 1. The different types of digital radiography

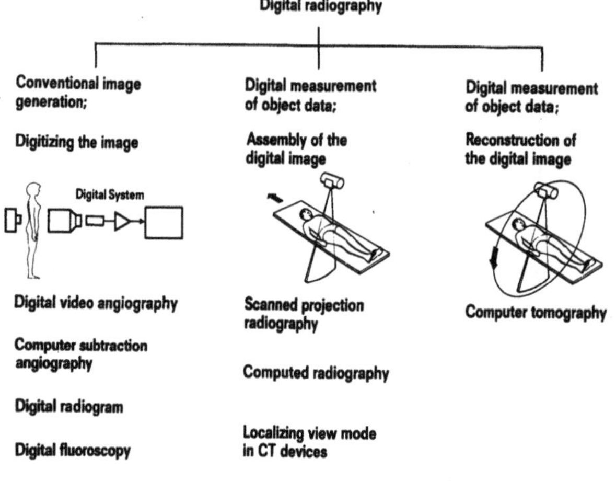

Fig. 2. Examples of digital radiography

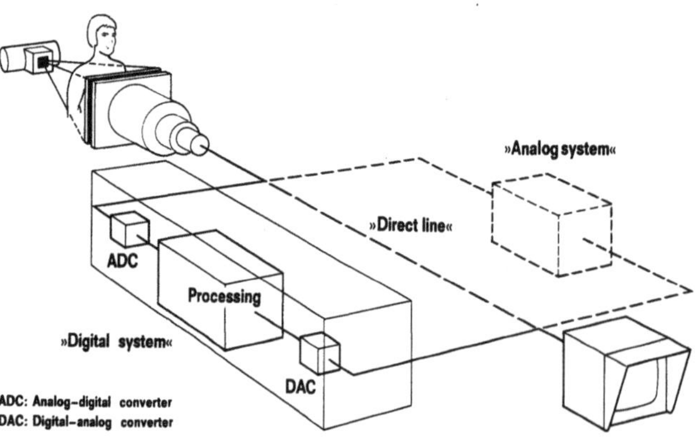

Fig. 3. Digital fluoroscopy and fluorographic system

	Analog	Digital
Limitations »for the best results« essentially given	by »practical physics«	by costs
Statement illustrated by: **Image data storage** regarding	**Video tape/disk** with	**Solid state memory** with
● Additional noise	Internal noise sources including drop-outs	*Quantization noise* depends upon *Bits per picture element*
● Spatial resolution losses	Finite gap width of write–read head	*fineness of matrix*, depends upon *picture elements per image*
● Quality decrease due to repeated storage	yes	no
Filtering, modification of gradation regarding	**Opto–electronical components** with	**Digital processor**
● Additional noise	Internal noise sources	As above
● Spatial resolution losses	Inhomogeneous and anisotropic transmission characteristics, e. g. parasitic capacitors	

Fig. 4. Essential differences between analog and digital imaging, recording and processing

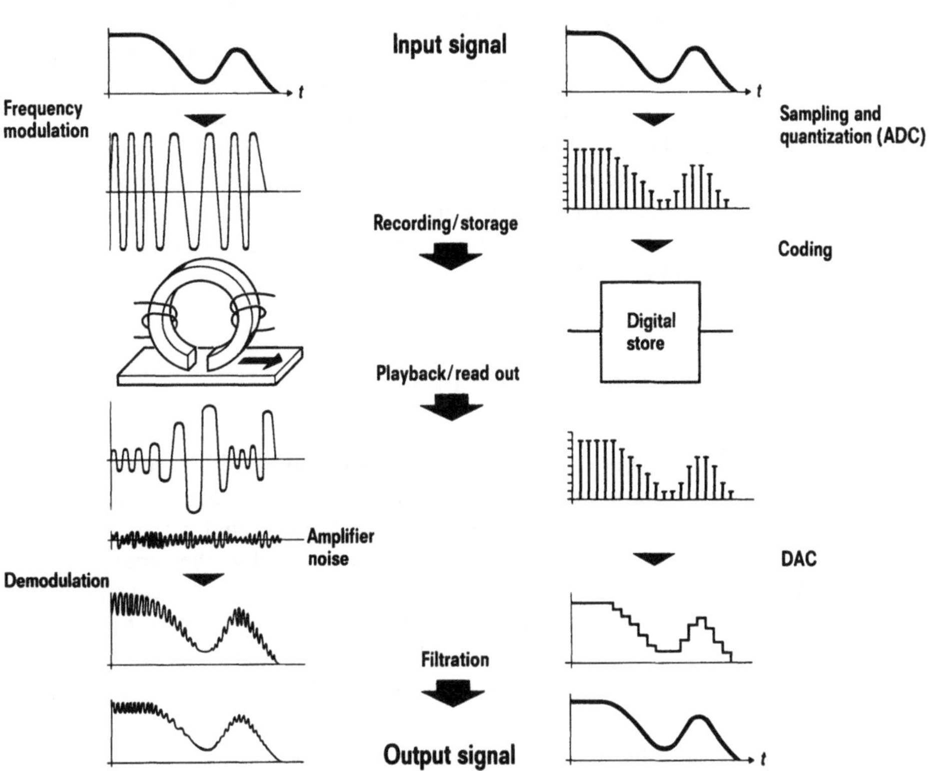

Fig. 5. Example for analog versus digital storage

values of the input signal the frequency of the intermediate signal is also high. When recording these signals on tape, the high-frequency magnetic fieds in the gap of the recording head change too quickly for the tape to be able to move over the head gap during a specific magnetic field change. Consequently, the magnetic field

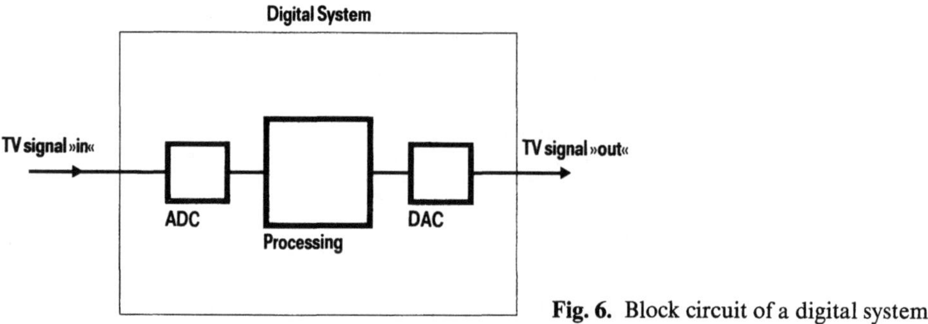

Fig. 6. Block circuit of a digital system

amplitude is 'smeared' over the tape. The signal is diminished when being recorded and when read during playback. Internal noise sources of the tape recording electronics have less effect on the large amplitudes than on the lesser amplitudes of higher modulation frequencies. Therefore, the demodulated playback video signal contains noise in proportion to its amplitude.

When storing digital signals, the situation is different. After the analog signal has been sampled ('temporal discretization'), each signal value has an integer allocated to it (amplitude quantization) which on being read out appears again as exactly this integer. This is a consequence of the yes-or-no reaction of the individual storage cells. Systematic errors may arise during the sampling process, i.e. how many samples should be taken per unit time and, during quantizing, to what degree of fineness should the amplitude steps be selected? These are questions of technical necessity and related cost.

2 Digital Components and Their Function

An analog signal is fed to the digital system as illustrated in Fig. 3, corresponding to an X-ray TV image. Before 'processing', i.e. further manipulation of the signal by digital means, the analog signal is converted into a digital signal capable of being read by digital electronics (Fig. 6). This is performed by the analog-digital converter (ADC) which interrogates the continuous analog signal (sampling) at regular intervals and allocates a discrete numerical value to it (quantization). Since only a limited supply of integers is available, e.g. from 0 to 255 ($\triangleq$ 8 Bit) for quantizing the analog signal, values must be allocated at the instance nearest to the actual values (Fig. 7).

The error which thereby arises is known as the quantizing error. In the ideal situation, it amounts to $\pm \frac{1}{2}$ amplitude step. The representation of the integer amplitude value obtained in this way, normally in binary form, is known as coding. When receiving signals from a TV system, the sampling frequency is determined by the size of the matrix chosen. With a matrix size of 256×256 picture elements (pixels) the ADC works with a sampling frequency of approximately 1.6 MHz. With a matrix of 512×512, a minimum frequency of 12.5 MHz is required. In actual practice, 20 MHz must be used, since the image signal does not occur

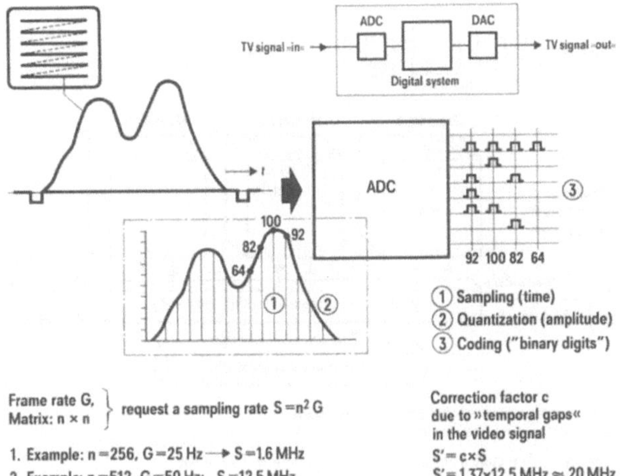

Fig. 7. Principle of analog-to-digital conversion

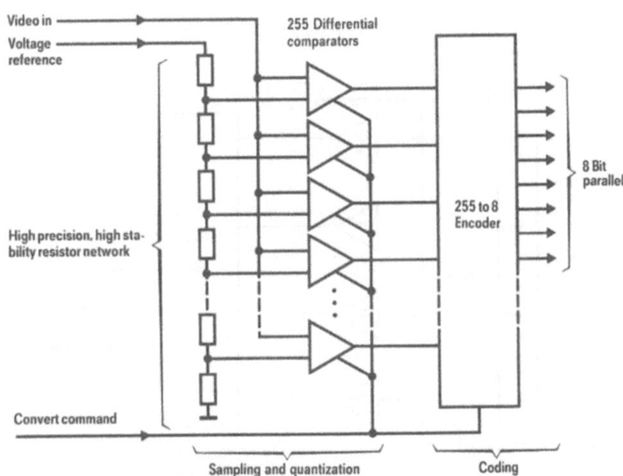

Fig. 8. Schematic of an 8 Bit video flash analog-to-digital converter

constantly during the image time but is interrupted by auxiliary signals used in TV technology, e.g. blanking intervals. The fineness of the amplitude quantization depends on the signal and its inherent exactness and on quantum noise.

Figure 8 demonstrates the principle of the ADC. First of all, with the aid of the comparators (voltage comparing networks) it is determined what value the analog signal has reached or exceeded. The comparators which respond to this signal ensure that the encoder transmits a 'Bit-pattern' corresponding to its value over the output leads, as a parallel-pulse signal. (in Fig. 7 for the mV values 92, 100, 82, 64 at the output of the ADC, the binary numbers 01011100, 01100100, 01010010, 01000000 are indicated.)

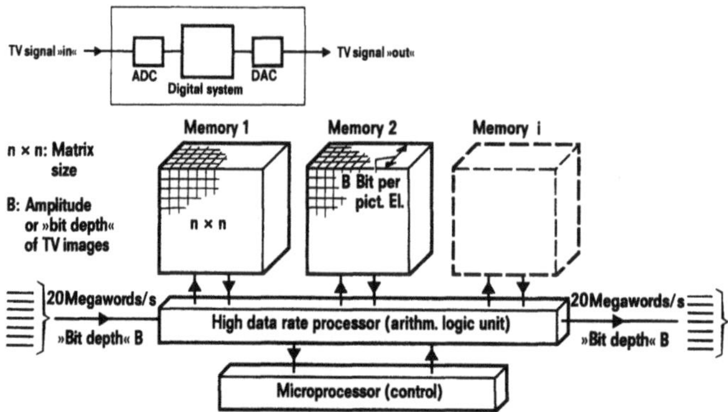

Fig. 9. Principal structure of a digital processing system

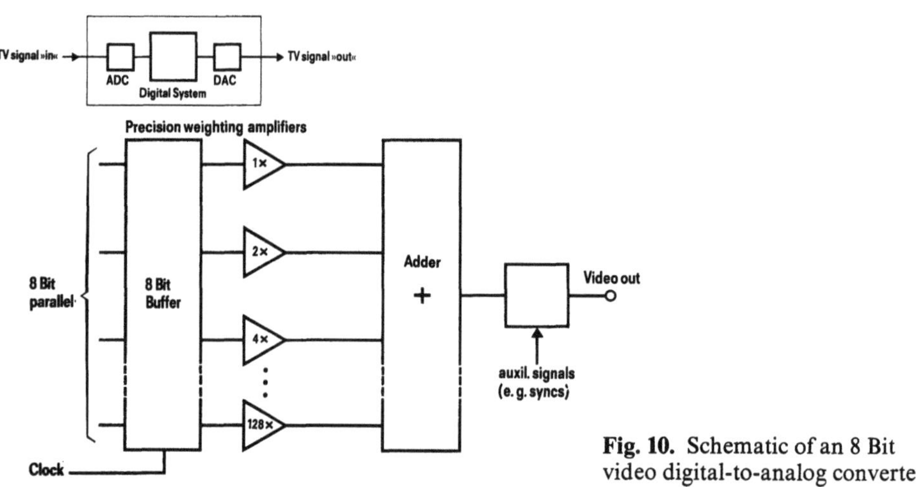

Fig. 10. Schematic of an 8 Bit video digital-to-analog converter

In the 'digital system' the operations take place as binary digital processes. Because of the high data throughput due to the high number of pixels per frame and the high frame rate of the TV system, the calculation processes are handled in a special processor through which the total data transport flows (Fig. 9) between the input and output of the digital system and to and from the main memories. One can conceive of these main memories as being image orientated, i.e. with a memory address number corresponding to the matrix size, in which under each address one pixel is filed, e.g. to the Bit depth 8 Bit or of a word length or 8 Bit. The microprocessor, unsuitable as a universal processor for the necessary rapid signal processing, takes over regulating and control duties, as also in the interactive mode with the system user. Figure 9 also shows how the system costs increase due to the number of expensive semiconductor memories if these memories are not used simultaneously for numerous images.

After the processing, there is only a binary coded TV signal. To display the results of the processing as an image, the digital signal must be reconverted into an analog video signal. This is performed by the digital-analog converter (DAC/ Fig. 10). The digits on the individual lines are converted into a part signal corresponding to the numerical value which they represent and these part signals are added. This process has already been demonstrated in Fig. 5, where the part signals are appropriately elongated to fill out the ADC sampling interval and the arising stepped form is smoothed out by analog low-pass filtering.

3 Digital Subtraction Angiography

3.1 System Build-Up

Regarding system performance, the box labelled 'processing' is the most important element (Fig. 6). In this the two image memories are allocated two tasks. At all events, the images for the angiographic subtraction process are stored in them, i.e. the subtraction of the 'natural image' or the 'mask' (temporal phase, before contrast medium opacification) from the 'opacified image' or angiogram proper. Needless to say, any other two phases of an angiographic examination, e.g. an arterial and venous phase, can be stored and subtracted from one another to result in a combined arteriovenous image. But prior to this, a series of successive TV images are integrated in each memory at its time of action by the aid of an arithmetic-logic unit (ALU). This integration is performed so that from a number of individual TV images, with, for example, the usual low fluoroscopic image dose and corresponding quantum noise proportion, a new image can be produced, with higher effective dose and thus better signal-to-noise ratio. The system presented lies in the X-ray TV chain (Fig. 3) without intervention in its image cycle (frame rate). From this system, first of all technical and then diagnostic advantages are to be derived. From the technical point of view, the expense of modifying the image cycle is eliminated, e.g. to two or three images per second and the inclusion of the generator that is therefore necessary in the control of the digital system. It is self-evident that in such a case the generator must work in the pulse mode: high pulse output to achieve individual images of low quantum noise is then indispensable.

From the diagnostic point of view, the summation of the sequential TV frames to achieve adequately low-noise individual images has the advantage of being able to review the period of contrast medium flow without any temporal gaps, in order to select the phase at which the opacification of the vessel was at an optimum. In the same way, it is possible to obtain a mask image directly before the opacification starts and since the length of time separating this from the image displaying the optimum opacification is the shortest; as a rule, the resulting subtraction image shows minimal motion artefacts.

The selection of such images, both within and without the opacification phase, is simplified by the subtraction fluoroscopic operation, in which a mask which has

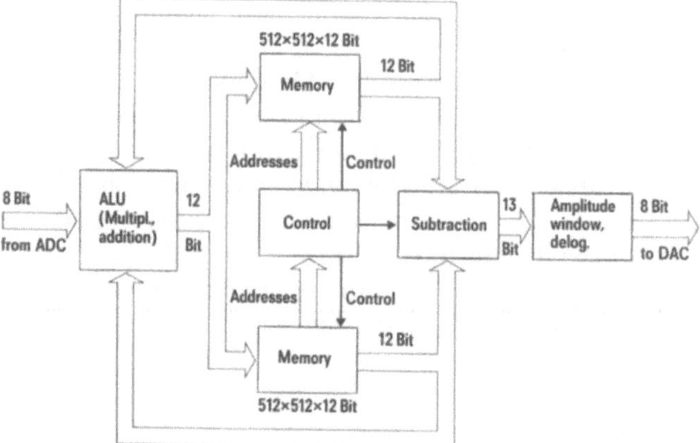

Fig. 11. Data flow in the digital system

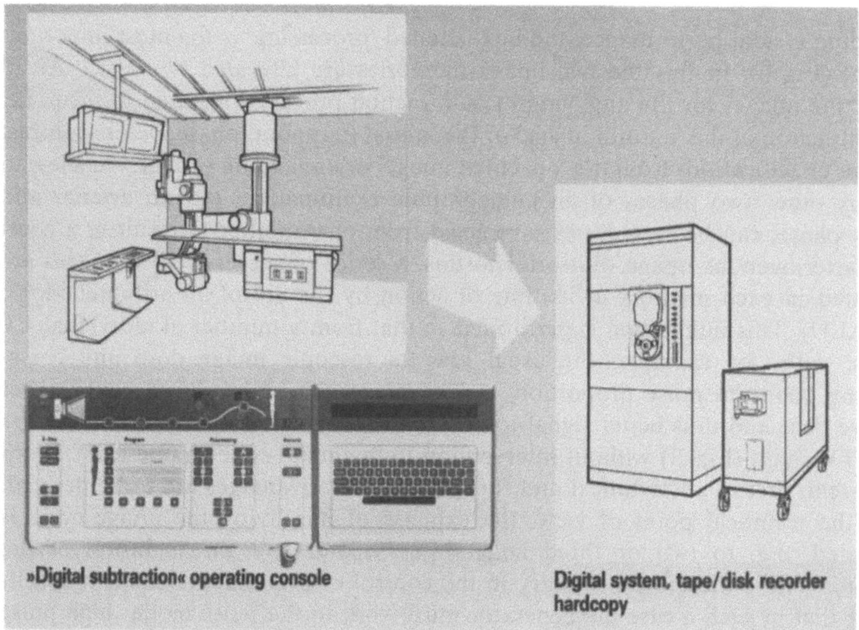

Fig. 12. Angiographic installation with digital subtraction system

been established at a specific time by the press of a button is continuously subtracted from ensuing fluoroscopic scenes. The subtraction fluoroscopic operation
should not, however, just be regarded as a convenient help in selecting optimum
phases. Because it is possible to observe the whole filling process in relation to time,
it acquires its own diagnostic significance.

Figure 12 again makes it clear that digital fluoroscopic subtraction angiography,
as a supplementary facility at an angiographic examination unit, brings with it no

special technical consequences for the fundamental X-ray installation. Tube assembly, generator and the image-intensifier TV system must naturally be lined up with one another for fluoroscopic subtraction, where, in itself, a high-resolution, high line-rate X-ray TV installation offers advantages in respect of image quality. In fluoroscopic subtraction, the second TV monitor has the task of displaying the subtraction-fluoroscopic images or exposures. The complete angiographic examination is recorded on video tape or by disc store, so that following the examination the desired subtraction phase can be produced in the replay mode and, in turn, documented by a hard-copy unit. From a user's viewpoint, the control console is the key item: To ensure problem-free integration into the examination procedure, operation must be simple and information feedbacks, e.g. on the subtraction results, must be fast and reliable. By means of the control panel shown here, the mask can be automatically recorded by timer initiation in relation to the injection, or alternately by push-button, and similarly, at a later point in time, the resulting opacified images are also established. In Fig. 11, at the output end of the system, a box is shown with the designation 'amplitude window' and 'Delog'. The selectable amplitude window has the task of modifying the amplitude range, so that it is favourable for optimum display of the contrast medium. The delogarithming is necessary so that the optional possibility of original image playback (mask or filling) can be displayed with the characteristics of a usual X-ray image which, of course, nobody is used to seeing in a logarithmic mode.

3.2 Component Characteristics

In fluoroscopic subtraction, besides the image subtraction itself, it is very important to integrate image packets or to determine the average of such a packet in order to obtain new individual images of higher effective dose and lower quantum noise. Figure 11 shows the two stores, in which this averaging process takes place with the aid of the ALU. Figure 13 shows a storage circuit as described by methods of communication theory (*Schüßler* 1973). The constants b_0 and c_0 of this 'recursive filter' have been selected such that

$$b_0 = \frac{1}{K} \quad \text{and} \quad c_0 = \frac{-(K-1)}{K}$$

in order that a continuous signal $U_i(k)$ and the signal $U_0(k)$ already contained in the intermediate store V can be summated to form a signal which at the maximum amplitudes of U_i and U_0 does not itself exceed this maximum amplitude, since

$$U_{max}\frac{1}{K} + U_{max}\frac{K-1}{K} = U_{max}$$

The output signal $U_0(k)$ in which k represents the numbering of the sampling intervals (in this case, the frame numbering of the TV system) can be given as a 'recursive formula' (Fig. 13, first line lower left), in which the intermediate memory functions as an element which repeats the signal reaching it, delayed by one sampling interval or one TV frame. If this equation is solved for U_0, the U_0 is seen as a function of all preceding image signals.

                                                                P. Marhoff and M. Pfeiler

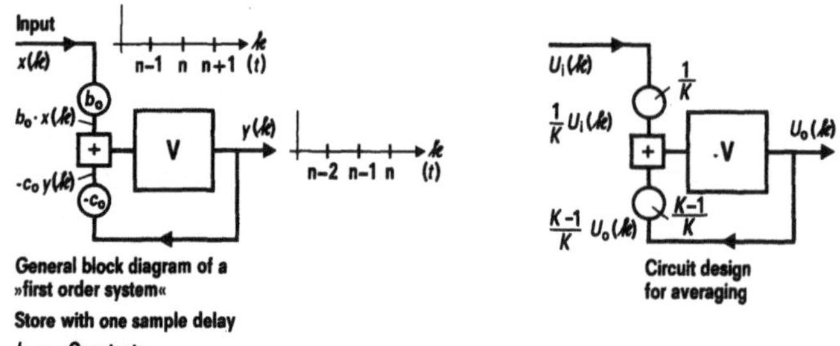

$$U_o(k)=V\left\{\frac{1}{K}\,U_i(k)+\frac{K-1}{K}\,U_o(k)\right\} \qquad U_o(k)=\frac{1}{K}\,U_i(k-1)+\frac{K-1}{K}\,U_o(k-1)$$

$$U_o(k)=\frac{1}{K}\left[U_i(k-1)+\frac{K-1}{K}\,U_i(k-2)+\left(\frac{K-1}{K}\right)^2 U_i(k-3)+\cdots\right]$$

Fig. 13. Storage circuit for averaging

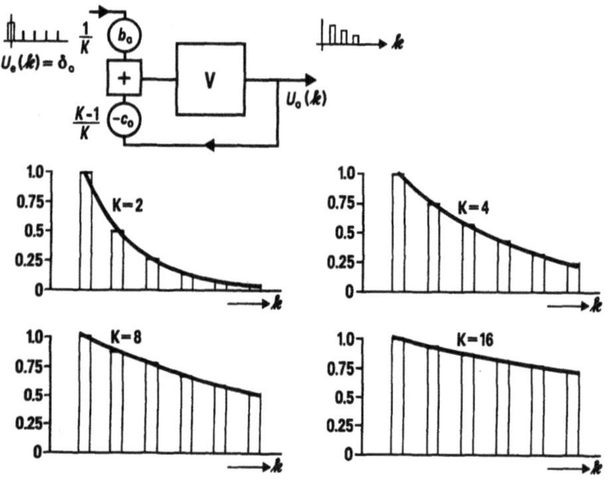

Fig. 14. Pulse response or weighting function of the storage circuit for averaging

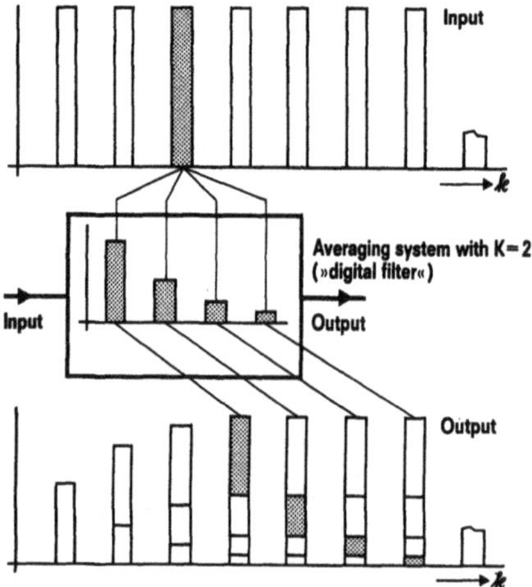

Fig. 15. Averaging the digitized signal sequence: Contribution of one input image to the sequence of output images

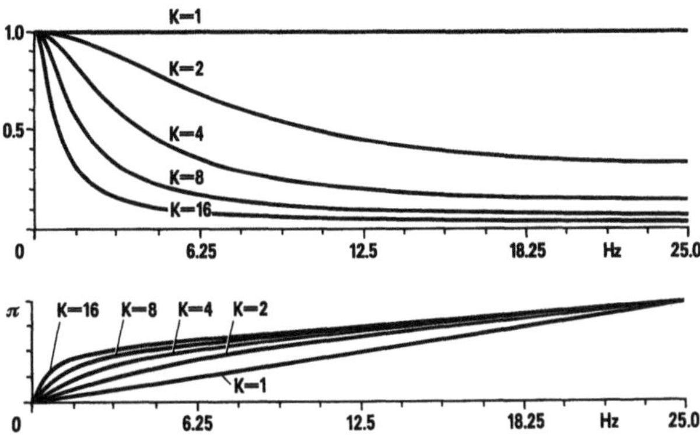

Fig. 16. Transfer function of the storage circuit for averaging. Corresponding to the pulse responses of the storage circuit (Fig. 14)

Besides this, it depends on the evaluation factor K to what extent the input signal values are included in the output signal. With an input signal consisting of one pulse, it is possible to obtain a very rapid overview (Fig. 14). When K is small, the effect of the input signal reduces relatively quickly; Fig. 15 shows an example with K = 2 and thus how from a series of input signals the individual signal influences the series of output signals. According to the curves in Fig. 14, for K = 2, the two input signals which have occurred immediately before have the most significant effect on an output signal. In fact, only K images out of an input sequence would have an effect on the output, if one were to proceed further in pulse response (Fig. 14) using only the evaluation factor 1/K in each case. Then the maximum amplitude of the output image signal would be reached with K image signals alone.

The block circuit diagram shown in Fig. 13 as a linear system can be assigned a transfer function equivalent to the pulse response, which Fig. 16 shows for various evaluation factors. Here, it can be seen that the integration or averaging of an increasing number of frames proportional to K results in a more or less characteristic low-pass filter behaviour. Thus, with K which determines the number of input images which form a sliding 'integration packet' and contribute to the output image, the effective dose of this output image can be selected.

In Fig. 17, the 'summation' or 'arithmetical averaging' is compared with the 'sliding average' described above. If only one memory is available, as in the case of the recursive system of the sliding average value determination, then the memory can only be filled by the start/stop method, that is to say, with a preselected number of images. A sliding of the image packeting and thus 'moving' integration, however, is not possible.

The signal-to-noise ratio improvements given in Fig. 17 are based on the following short calculation. For the 'arithmetical averaging' or summation of K individual images to a resulting image of equal signal amplitude, in which n_0 quanta contribute to an individual image point, for the noise (RMS – Root Mean Square – amplitude) in the individual image one can write:

$$N_K = \text{const } \sqrt{n_0}$$

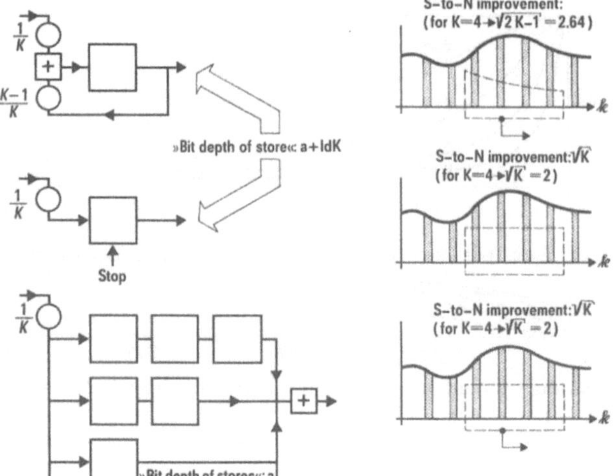

Fig. 17. Digital averaging and summation

where const. is the system parameter. The resulting noise is the geometric mean of the individual noise signal N_k, thus:

$$N = \frac{1}{K}\sqrt{K \cdot N_K^2} = \frac{1}{K}\sqrt{K \cdot \text{const}^2 \, n_0} = \text{const}\sqrt{\frac{n_0}{K}} \, .$$

In respect of N_k there is thus an improvement of

$$\frac{N}{N_K} = \frac{1}{\sqrt{K}} \, .$$

The signal-to-noise ratio (with the signal remaining constant) thus improves by $\sqrt{K}$. In this calculation, it is assumed that signal and noise are exclusively due to the statistics of the X-ray quanta and that this noise is statistically independent, and from frame to frame a TV camera tube without lag is assumed.

Under the same conditions, from the relationship shown in Fig. 13, the reduction of the noise or the improvement of the signal-to-noise ratio is derived for an image produced by sliding or weighted averaging. Again, with the same type of individual images, each of which is built up from n_0 quanta, for the signal S, as the weighted sum of the individual signals, there results:

$$S = \frac{1}{K}S_K\left(1 + \frac{K-1}{K} + \left(\frac{K-1}{K}\right)^2 + \left(\frac{K-1}{K}\right)^3 + \ldots\right)$$

or, according to the summation formula of the infinite geometrical series:

$$S = \frac{1}{K} \cdot \frac{1}{1 - \dfrac{K-1}{K}} = S_K \, .$$

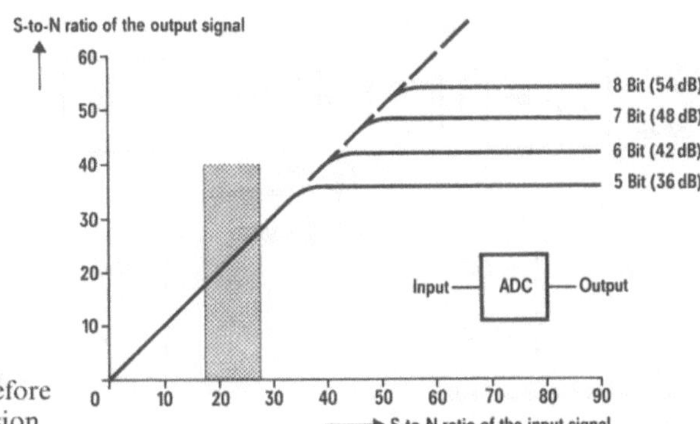

Fig. 18. Signal-to-noise ratio before and after analog-to-digital conversion

For the noise, the contributions of the individual images are again added geometrically, thus:

$$N = \frac{1}{K} N_K \sqrt{1 + \left(\frac{K-1}{K}\right)^2 + \left(\frac{K-1}{K}\right)^4 + \dots}$$

or

$$N = \frac{1}{K} N_K \sqrt{\frac{1}{1 - [(K-1)/K]^2}} = \text{const} \sqrt{n_0} \sqrt{\frac{1}{2K-1}}.$$

The signal-to-noise ratio thus improves by $2K - 1$.

In respect of an improvement of the signal-to-noise ratio (thus, reduction of the noise, measured at the signal), there is a slight advantage for the sliding averaging, since here, for $K = 4$, a signal-to-noise ratio is obtained, improved by the factor 2.64, whereas the arithmetical averaging yields a factor of only 2. However, it must be considered that for these mathematical derivations it is assumed that the signal defined for subtraction angiography (the contrast medium) is uniformly present in all individual images, since an infinitely long image sequence contributes to the sliding averaging. For rapid changes of the concentration of the contrast medium, for example, those that are shorter than the time for 16 images (i.e. $16 \cdot 20$ ms $= 0.31$ s) in respect of the 'effective' signal-to-noise ratio, the arithmetical averaging could be the most favourable. Should this also be carried out by the "sliding" method, which seems indispensable in clinical procedure, then this would mean an outlay in the example selected, for $(K(K-1))/2$ memory units.

It is evident that in the case of averaging with only one memory it must be capable of accepting an input signal reduced by the evaluation factor K, i.e. the ratio of the smallest to the largest signal value occurring in the memory, or its dynamic range, is to be set larger than the Bit depth or amplitude resolution of the original signal by the factor K. Thus, the amplitude resolution of the memory increases by ld K Bit in comparison to the amplitude resolution 'a' of the ADC. If the case $K = 16$ is considered, the memory has to have 4 Bit more than the ADC; therefore, in the case in point 12 Bit are necessary.

The question remains whether the 8 Bit or amplitude resolution of the ADC is sufficient for an adequately exact signal transmission. The curves in Fig. 18 show the additional interference (noise) with which the output signal is encumbered in

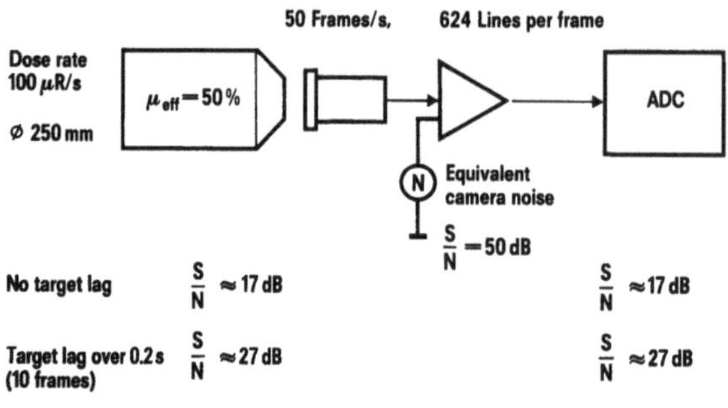

Fig. 19. Signal-to-noise ratio in the image intensifier television chain

comparison with the input signal, in accordance with the Bit depth of the ADC (*Paulson* 1979). The relationship signal to interference (noise) is expressed in dB (decibels) and for the signal-to-noise ratio S/N the relationship

$$\frac{S}{N} = 20 \log \frac{\text{Signal amplitude (Peak-to-Peak)}}{\text{RMS noise}} \text{ dB}$$

applies. It is possible to conceive the origination of the curves in the following manner: With ideally fine quantization by the ADC, the magnitude at its input undergoes no change and, in this ideal case, the signal-to-noise ratio is reproduced; represented in the diagram by the 45° straight line through the origin. With a finite Bit depth and an input signal without or with only slight noise, i.e. with a large signal-to-noise ratio, in an unfavourable case an uncertainty of half a step occurs in the output signal. In the case of the 8 Bit ADC, this means that with a full signal, that is, one which encompasses 256 steps, there is a signal-to-noise ratio of

$$\frac{S}{N} = \frac{1}{2} \frac{1}{256},$$

or expressed in decibels

$$\frac{S}{N} = 20 \log, \ \frac{1}{512} = 54 \text{ dB}.$$

Thus, the second asymptote to the signal-to-noise ratio curve is given. The quantization error brought about by the ADC, cannot be designated as noise in the usual sense; with an unchanged input signal, the quantization error included in the output signal also remains constant.

An assessment will now be made, as to how large the signal-to-noise ratio of the analog signal is which arises in the X-ray TV chain, in order to establish whether and to what degree an ADC with 8 Bit is adequate.

If one assumes the following data, as shown in Fig. 19:

– Diameter of the image intensifier input field: 25 cm
– Effective quantum absorption: η eff = 50%
– 500 lines per frame, at 50 frames/s
– Number of quanta per dose
  (diagnostic radiation quality): $2.4 \times 10^4 + \dfrac{\text{quanta}}{\mu\text{R cm}^2}$,

then with the pixel height of 250 mm/500 = 0.5 mm and an assumed equally wide pixel width, there is a signal-to-noise ratio of less than 20 dB, when the dose rate at the image intensifier input is 100 µR/s, even in the case of a TV camera tube showing some lag.

The sampling frequency of the signals was already set at 20 MHz, in accordance with Fig. 7, so that in line with the sampling theorem of the electrical communication theory, the video amplifier is limited to 10 MHz in its bandwidth (with the steepest possible filter flank, in order to use optimally the good contrast performance of the existing 25 MHz amplifier). Under these conditions, for the TV camera alone, there is a signal-to-noise ratio of more than 50 dB (also related to the maximum signal or full modulation). Thus, the additional noise from the camera amplifier is negligibly small compared with the quantum noise and it remains small even if the signal-to-noise ratio assigned to the X-rays were to increase to more than 40 dB. At 40 dB, the signal-to-noise ratio would still lie substantially below the limiting characteristics of the 8 Bit ADC; thus, the dose rate could – in respect of the ADC – be without problems up to the factor 10, in the case of a camera tube with lag, or by the factor 100 in the case of a lag-free camera tube.

However, in Fig. 19, it has not been taken into consideration that between the incoming video signal and the ADC there is a logarithmation unit for the extraction of the attenuation value signal. The 'logarithmic characteristic' of this unit is still to be dealt with. It has an effect on the signal-to-noise ratio of the ADC incoming signal, since the logarithmic characteristic curve in the area of full modulation improves the signal-to-noise ratio of the video signal; there again, in the case of small modulations, it is made worse. With a two-decade logarithmation unit, at full modulation an improvement of

$$\frac{1}{\frac{\log e}{2}}, \quad \text{that is 13.3 dB,}$$

is to be expected, but at minimum modulation, it is made worse by

$$\frac{1}{100\frac{\log e}{2}}, \quad \text{that is 53.3 dB.}$$

Thus, with extremely high signal values, the reserve area of the dose rate addressed by the logarithmation unit (factor 10 or 100) is narrowed by 20%, which is practically nothing, but with small modulations (object area with higher attenuation in comparison to the surroundings) the improvement extends considerably above this reserve.

Respecting the subtraction itself, it should be mentioned that the image signals (mask and filling phase) provided for the subtraction should be available fundamentally as logarithmated intensity signals (Fig. 20), if, up to the signal changes brought about by the contrast medium, otherwise absolutely identical images (i.e. exactly the same exposure conditions) are to be subtracted from one another. In 'linear' subtraction, with the same contrast medium concentration, the result of the

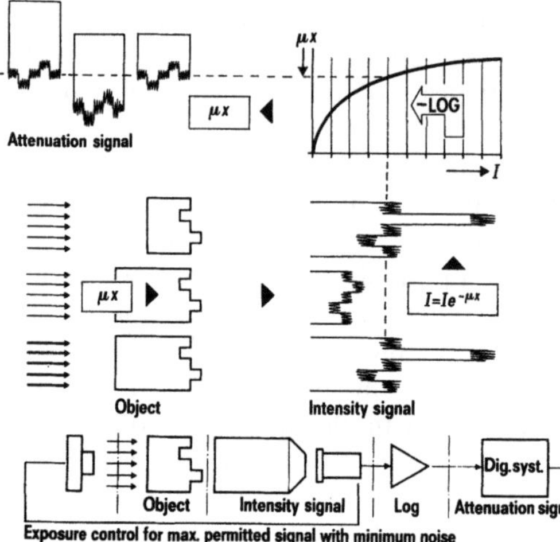

Fig. 20. Transformation of the intensity signal into the attenuation signal by logarithms before analog-to-digital conversion

subtraction depends on the intensity at a given position, i.e. from the tissue properties (density, thickness, material) which exist there. Suppose, for instance, in the simplest case of homogeneous tissue and monochromatic radiation, at a given position in the mask image I_M is such that:

$$I_M = I_0\, e^{-\mu d}$$ (where μ is the attenuation coefficient and d is the tissue thickness),

then by the substitution of a tissue layer having the thickness Δ by a contrast medium of attenuation coefficient μ_K in the filling image, there would be the intensity I_K, such that:

$$I_K = I_0\, e^{-[\mu(d-\Delta)+\mu_K\Delta]} = I_M\, e^{-(\mu_K-\mu)\Delta}\,.$$

In the subtraction image, the signal would thus be:

$$I_S = I_K - I_M = I_M\,[e^{-(\mu_K-\mu)\Delta} - 1]$$

and therefore dependent on the "base signal" I_M.

In comparison, the difference L_S of the logarithmated signals is

$$L_S = \log I_K - \log I_M = \log e\,(\mu - \mu_K)\,\Delta$$

where $\log e = 0.43$, thus independent of the base signal or the nature and thickness of the tissue to be contrasted.

Now, the logarithmation only yields the desired "linearization in μd" approximately, for in fact the X-rays are polychromatic. Therefore, as a consequence of the dependence of the subtraction on the base signal, residual errors are to be expected and become evident, e.g. as loss of contrast in opacified vessels at points where bone structures are crossed (hardening-up effect). A similar effect can be ascribed to the scattered radiation. Both influences and the possibility of compensating for them are being discussed (*Riederer* et al. 1981).

It remains to be said that for the practical operation of the system presented in the block circuit diagram, the radiation power always has to be adjusted by an

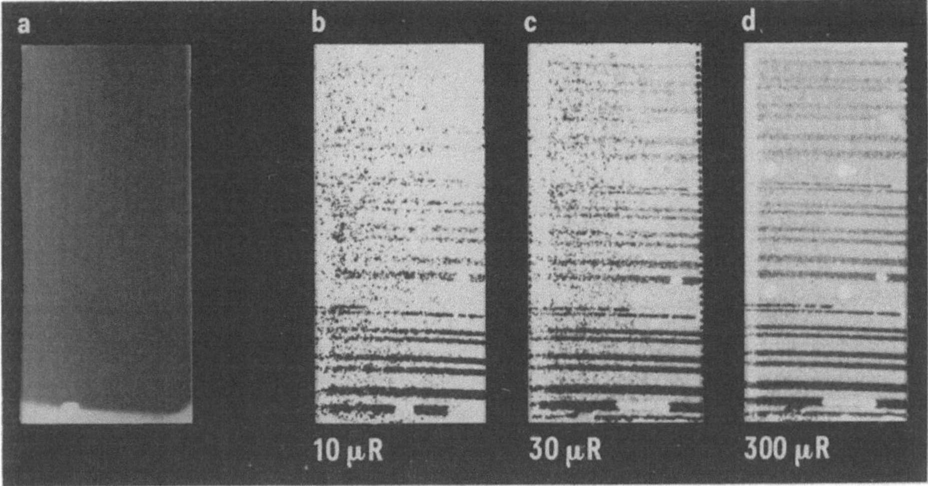

Fig. 21 a–d. Filling and subtraction images of an object phantom (aluminium steps with contrast medium structure superimposed), with varying image dose. **a** Filling exposure; **b, c, d** subtraction images at 70 kV. Evaluation factor K = 16

automatic exposure device, so that the intensity behind the object, measured via a dominant, remains constant. Thus, the greatest number of quanta are always available for the image, i.e. the greatest possible signal-to-noise ratio is attained. In order that this is only to the advantage of the diagnostically interesting region, the maximum intensity should occur there: The occurrence of 'free" radiation must be absolutely avoided by correct collimation.

4 Results and Discussion

With reference to the foregoing deliberations, in this section the results of image experiments with object phantoms are demonstrated.

Figure 21 a shows the fluoroscopic stored image of aluminium steps with an object range (ratio of the intensity from behind the first step to behind the last step) of 15 : 1. Arranged behind the steps is a Plexiglas plate with slots filled with contrast medium (corresponding to the 'filling image' in subtraction angiography) which can be moved by a motor so that a similar Plexiglas plate, but in this case without contrast medium, takes its place (corresponding to the 'empty image' or 'mask' in subtraction angiography). The examples b, c and d represent subtraction images. The increasing effective image dose from left to right was achieved by increasing the dose rate. The images were obtained in fluoroscopic operation. For all images, the evaluation factor for determining the average value was selected at K = 16. As would be ecpected, under otherwise equivalent conditions the noise drops dramatically, and even fine contrast medium structures are clearly recognizable. The contrast medium fillings of various widths shown in pairs are collected into groups of dif-

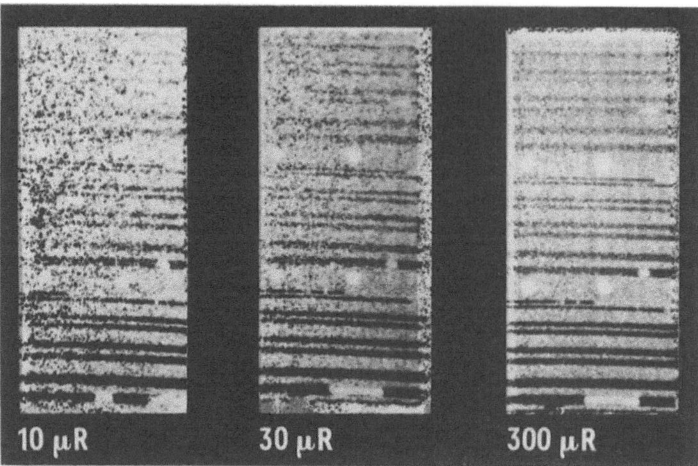

Fig. 22. Subtraction images as in Fig. 21 but with video tape intermediate storage of the angiographic scene

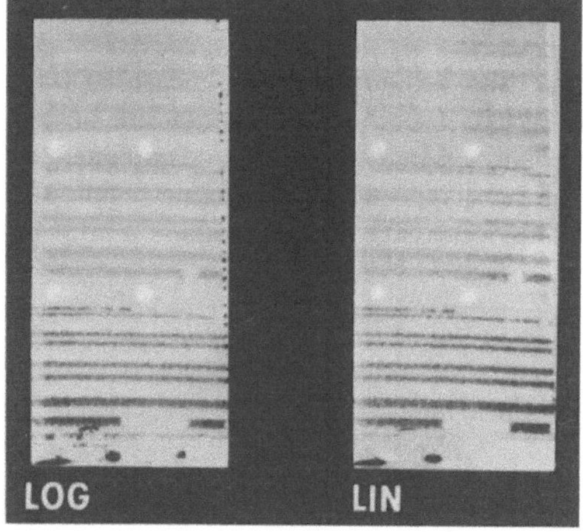

Fig. 23. Subtraction images of the object phantom, in accordance with Fig. 22, but with and without logarithmation. *Right,* the 'linear case' with basic attenuation-dependent blackening of the contrast medium structure

ferent concentration which correspond to an intensity change in the radiation image of approximately 1%, 2% and 5%.

The visible defects in the paths of the contrast medium (seen especially clearly in the image with the highest dose value) are due to the non-uniform distribution of the contrast medium, e.g. by sedimentation.

Figure 22 shows subtractions which differ from those in Fig. 21 only in that they were not obtained during a live fluoroscopic scene, so to say 'on-line', but were produced by the subsequent 'off-line' processing of a fluoroscopic recording by a video recorder. The additionally effective noise due to the intermediate magnetic

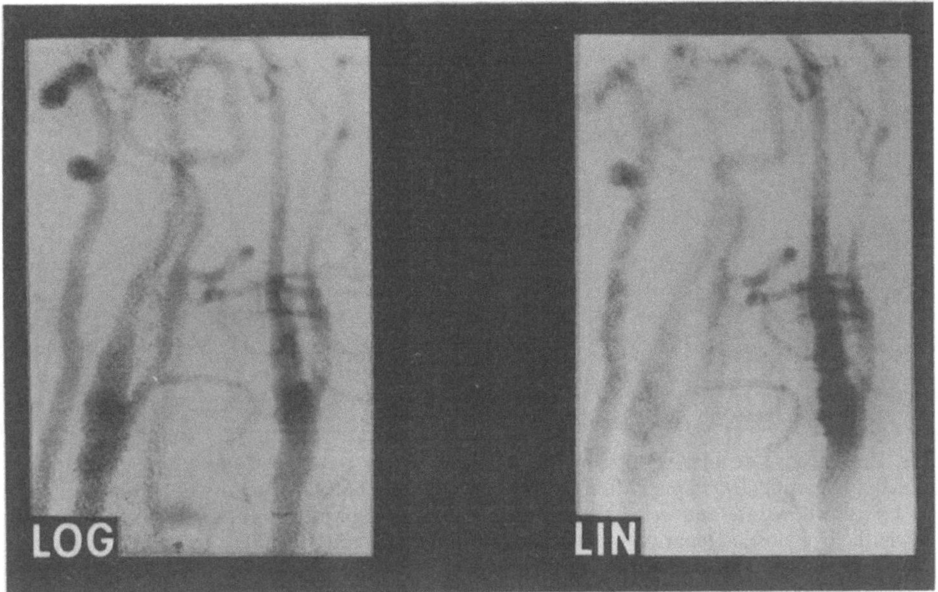

Fig. 24. Subtraction images from an intravenous angiography with and without logarithmation. Courtesy of Dr. W Seyferth, Diagnostic Department, Radiology Centre (Director Prof. Dr. E. Zeitler), Klinikum Nuremberg, D-8500 Nuremberg

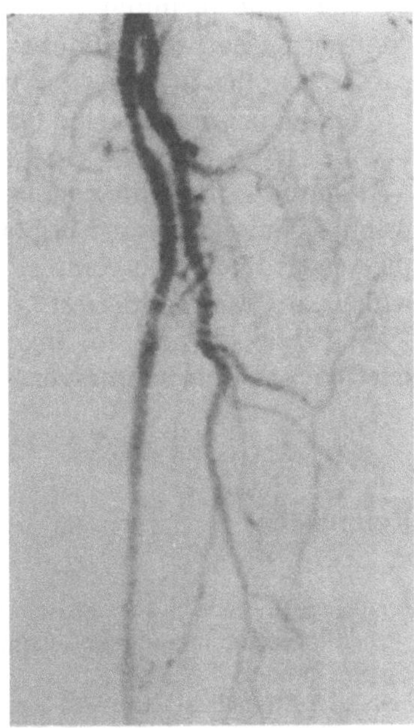

Fig. 25. Digital subtraction angiography demonstrating the superficial and deep femoral arteries following intravenous injections of 40 ml contrast material. Courtesy of Dr. W Seyferth, Diagnostic Department, Radiology Centre (Direktor Prof. Dr. E. Zeitler), Klinikum Nuremberg, D-8500 Nuremberg

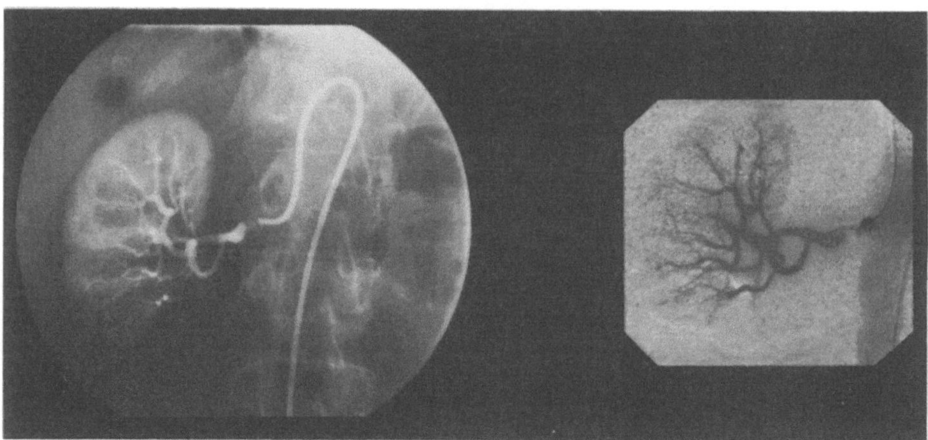

Fig. 26. Selective renal angiography. *Right,* renal artery stenosis. Comparison of a conventional angiogram (100 mm spotfilm) with one using only half the quantity of contrast medium at half the flow rate and using the subtraction image digital technique. Courtesy of Dr. W. Seyferth, Diagnostic Department, Radiology Centre, (Director Prof. Dr. E. Zeitler), Klinikum Nuremberg, D-8500 Nuremberg

recording can indeed be recognized, but it represents no significant loss of image quality.

The same phantom was also used for the subtraction images in Fig. 23 to confirm the statement about logarithmation at the end of the preceding section. It can be seen that in 'linear' subtraction images with increasing basic attenuation due to the aluminium steps, the blackening of the 'vessels filled with contrast medium' becomes less.

Figure 24 shows the comparison between 'linear' and 'logarithmic' subtraction, using a clinical example displaying the carotid arteries: Without logarithmation, the vessels filled with contrast medium would have been shown over their length with greatly varying contrast.

For Figs. 25 and 26, images from two medical case examples have been selected: one from an intravenous and one from a selective arterial angiography.

References

Brennecke R, Brown TK, Bürsch J, Heintzen PH (1976) Digital processing of videoangiocardiographic image series. Computers in Cardiology, IEEE Catalog No 76 CH 1160–1 C, pp 255–260

Feist JH, Sternglass EJ (1970) Application of TV subtraction techniques to clinical fluorographic procedures. Phys Med Biol 15:182

Frost MM, Fisher HD, Nudelman S, Roehrig H (1977) A digital video acquisition system for extraction of subvisual information in diagnostic medical imaging. SPIE, vol 127, Optical Instrumentation in Medicine VI, pp 208–215

Groh F (1967) Ein elektronisches Subtraktionsgerät. Roentgenpraxis 20:43–51

Mistretta CA, Kruger RA, Houk TL, Riederer SM, Shaw CG, Ergun D, Kubal W, Crummy AB, Zwiebel W, Rowe G, Zarnstorff W, Flemming D (1978) Computerized fluoroscopy techniques for non-invasive cardiovascular imaging. SPIE vol 152, Recent and Future Developments in Medical Imaging pp 65–71

Mistretta CA, Crummy AB, Strother CM (1981) Digital angiography: a perspective. Radiology 139:273–276

Paulson B (1979) Television is moving fast from A to D. Broadcast Communications, Sept 1979, pp 26–49

Riederer SJ, Pelc NJ, Georges J-PJ, Keyes GS, Lehmann LA, Hall AL (1981) Beam hardening, noise, and contrast considerations in selective Iodine digital radiography. IEEE Trans on Nucl Sci 28:pp 213–218

Schüßler HW (1973) Digitale Systeme zur Signalverarbeitung. Springer, Berlin Heidelberg New York

Ziedses des Plantes BG (1935) Subtraktion. Eine röntgenographische Methode zur separaten Abbildung bestimmter Teile des Objekts. ROEFO 52:69–79

Digital Radiography

M. P. Capp, S. Nudelman, D. Fisher, T. W. Ovitt, G. D. Pond,
M. M. Frost, H. Roehrig, J. Seeger and D. Oimette[1]

1 Introduction

In 1973, at the University of Arizona, we began an investigation into the role of
photoelectronic radiology in clinical medicine. Our goal was to look into the
possibility of replacing all x-ray film. At that time we had data, through the space
program, which showed that sophisticated television images were approaching the
detail found on x-ray films. However, we knew the system for replacement was not
ready and we asked ourselves if there was any component of it that could be
clinically applicable. We addressed the problem of imaging the vascular system in
this way. We used the conventional technique of film subtraction and applied it
digitally (*Roehrig* et al. 1976). Figure 1 demonstrates the very first successful
computerized subtracted image of carotid arteries in a dog, (1976). It should be
mentioned that at about the same time the University of Wisconsin under Mistretta
(*Kruger* et al. 1978, 1979), working independently, was also successful in developing
a system to carry out intravenous video subtraction. Our intravenous video subtraction images in patients started in our research laboratory in 1977 and in March
of 1980 we opened up a biplane special procedures room dedicated only toward
photoelectronic imaging (*Christenson* et al. 1980; *Ovitt* et al. 1980) (no film). This
has been quite successful and clinical examples will be shown later. Current efforts
are underway toward achieving total replacement of film. This is an immense
problem, one that will require a much greater sophistication of computers, storage
devices, systems analysis and great cooperation from both the radiologist and the
clinician (*Roehrig* et al. 1981). We theoretically converted our 70 000 procedures
per year department to complete photoelectronic imaging (no film). We estimated
that we would save approximately 5 million dollars over 10 years (*Nudelman* et al.,
to be published). Extrapolating this to the entire United States would result in a
conservative estimate of saving 1 billion dollars per year. Not included in these
mathematics are the cost-effective savings of all the time and effort of the
physicians.

---

1 The Department of Radiology, The University of Arizona, College of Medicine,
Tucson, AZ/USA

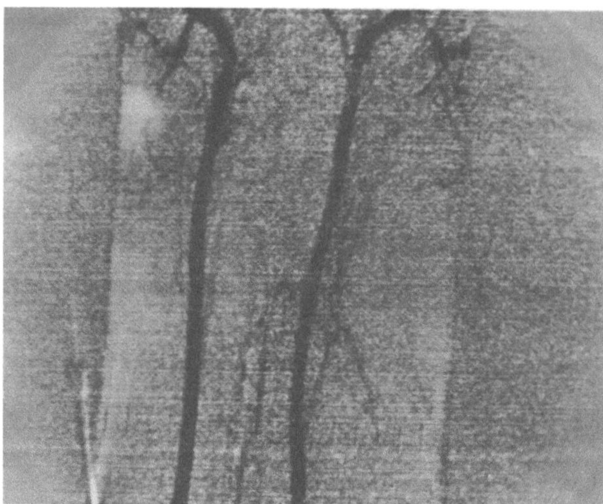

Fig. 1. This is the subtracted digital image with contrast enhancement of a dog and was produced in 1976. We were impressed with the excellent visualization of the carotid arteries

2 Methods

We have studied approximately 500 patients. These studies were virtually all performed on an outpatient basis by inserting a number 16 angiocath into the antecubital vein and, using the Seldinger technique, by advancing a 7 French catheter into the superior vena cava. Approximately 40 cc Renografin 76 are injected over 2 s and exposures are made at the rate of one per second for about 15 s.

Figure 2 demonstrates the system block diagram of our current system. The input dose to the image intensifier is about 1–1½ milliroentgens per frame or about 150 milliroentgens per exposure skin dose to the patient. We have used a 9-inch, 6-inch image intensifier, and on rare occasions a 4-inch. We plan to replace it by a special 16-inch and 9-inch CGR intensifer to handle the high exposure levels better and to give a larger area of exposure. The output of the intensifier is coupled to the video camera. The analog signal is then put through an A–D converter. The digitized video signal is fed in real time to a $512 \times 512 \times 8$ bit memory and from there very qucikly to the VAX 11-780 processing facility. A minimum of two pictures is necessary for intravenous angiography, one before the injection and one after the injection. The computer then performs a linear or logarithmic subtraction of the two images. The differential image is then enhanced in contrast using a digital "density window" and displayed on the high resolution CRT. For dynamic imaging, such as is necessary for blood flow or cardiac pulsations, the digitized video goes to a high density 130 digital tape recorder which can record up to 21 600 frames of $512 \times 512 \times 13$ bit video in real time.

It is important to point out that this is a rather complex system which is designed to do research on photoelectronic imaging devices in order to find

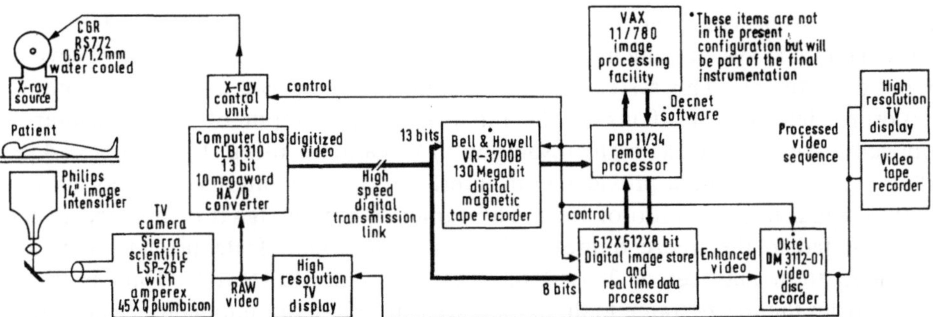

Fig. 2. This is a system block diagram representing the photoelectronic Department of Radiology at the University of Arizona. This system is quite sophisticated and obviously very expensive. From this system was devised a much more simple, inexpensive system shown in Fig. 3

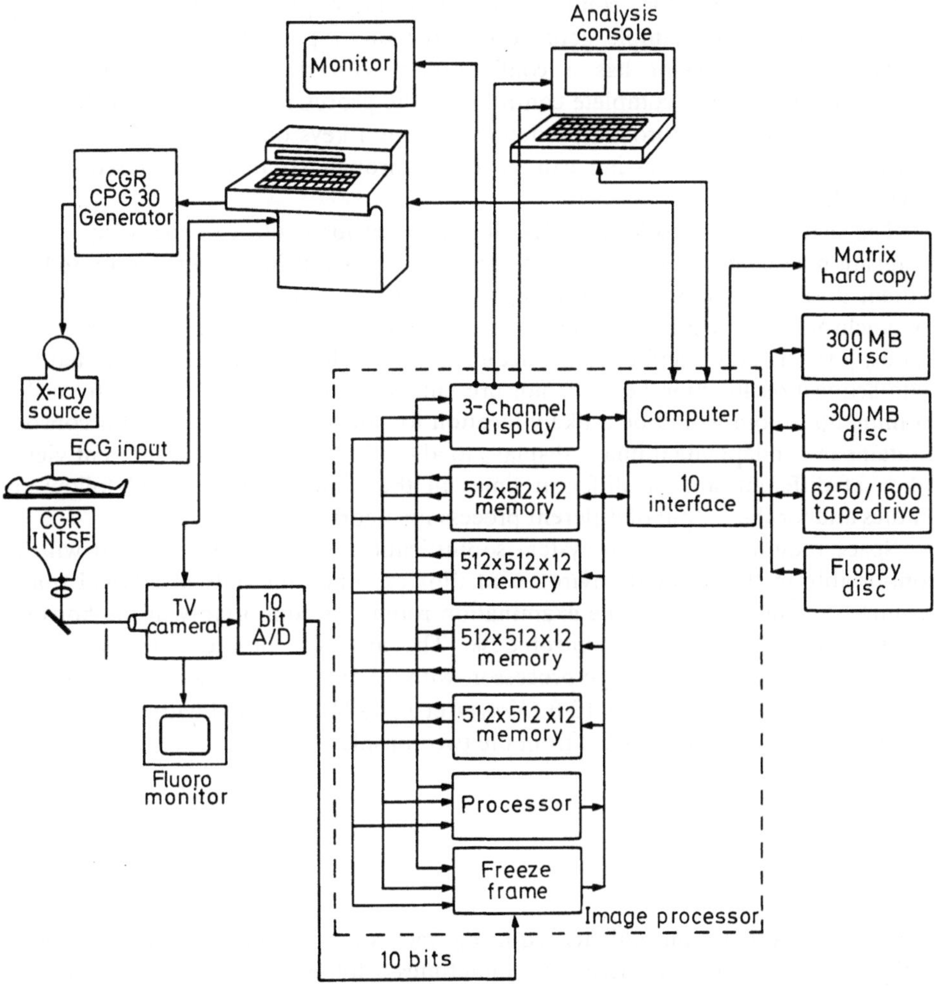

Fig. 3. This is a simplified, inexpensive, commercially available digital intravenous angiographic system (CGR) that was developed at the University of Arizona

optimum system components. Figure 3 demonstrates the phototype model of the CGR (DIVAS) system which at the time of printing will be operational in several x-ray departments. This system has the capability of stopping motion with one mr exposure delivered in 10 ms at the intensifier. The output of the intensifier is optically coupled to a high resolution TV camera using the Ampex 45× Plumbicon. The camera provides both interlaced and noninterlaced video formats with a signal to noise ratio of 1000. The camera's output signal is digitized to ten bits and fed to the freeze frame in the image processor. Data pixel formats are provided from matrices of 256×256; 512×512; and 1024×1024. Data is transferred from the freeze frame to digital memory in 1/30 s. Simultaneously, the digital data is transferred to a 300 megabyte disc at rates of up to three frames per second. Raw data can be viewed instantly; it can also be recalled for analysis in the image processor at the completion of the procedure. Most image analysis functions including subtraction, filtering, contrast stretching, averaging and magnification are performed in 1/30 s. More complicated algorithms require more time depending upon complexity, for example, geometric correction for patient motion.

The image processor has a configuration with three independent display channels. The user has complete control over the processing environment. Routine functions are initiated through predefined function keys on either of the consoles. More sophisticated processing can be done through commands entered at the keyboard.

The acquisition console provides the interface for control of the x-ray image acquisition system. This includes programmable acquisition patterns to reduce patient dose and data storage. It accepts an EKG gate to reduce patient motion or to synchronize for cardiac studies. The analysis console has the same keyboard, knobs, joystick, and interface as the acquisition console, with the exception that the data acquisition function keys are not present. A "reading room" remote from the examination room would be a likely location for the analysis console. This console contains two independent image displays to allow for comparison of different views taken at different studies, different times in the same study, pre and follow-up studies and/or the output of different processing algorithms.

Space required for all this system sophistication is quite reasonable. It will fit comfortably in the hospital environment. For example, the only additional space required for the controls at the examination room, fits comfortably in the housing provided for the generator control desk. The analysis console is the size of a standard office desk. The image processor, with all of its peripherals, can be placed in a room with an area of 10×10 ft (*Kruger* et al. 1978 d), located within a coupling electrical cable length of 300 feet from the two consoles.

3 Results

Neurological disease: all patients requiring neck studies have intravenous angiography and about 90% are successful. Sometimes a follow-up study for intracranial cerebral blood flow is done which has also been very helpful. Figure 4 demonstrates an occlusion of the right internal carotid artery. Since opening up our digital

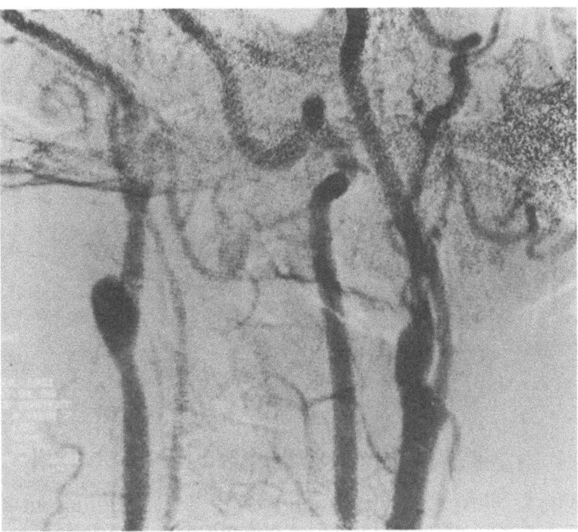

Fig. 4. This is an intravenous video subtraction angiogram demonstrating complete occlusion of the right internal carotid artery

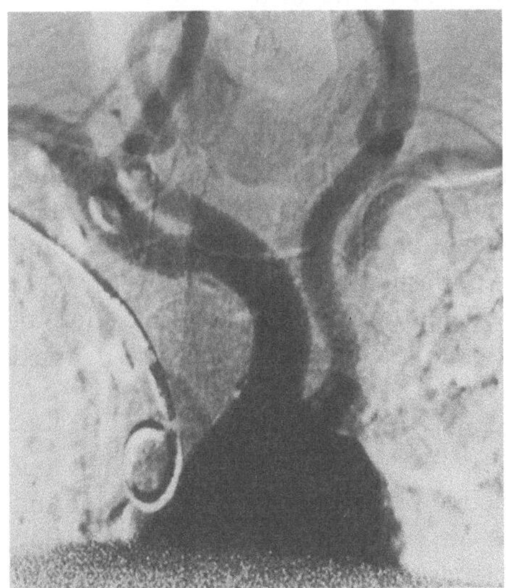

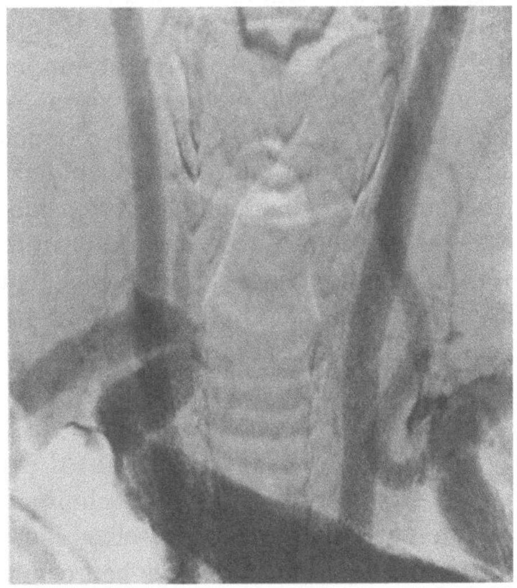

Fig. 5   **Fig. 6**

Fig. 5. This is a patient demonstrating complete occlusion of the left subclavian artery with subsequent filling of the subclavian by way of the steal phenomenon

Fig. 6. This is an intravenous subtraction angiogram demonstrating an anomalous right sucvlacian artery. The white area between the two carotids demonstrates a swallowing artifact

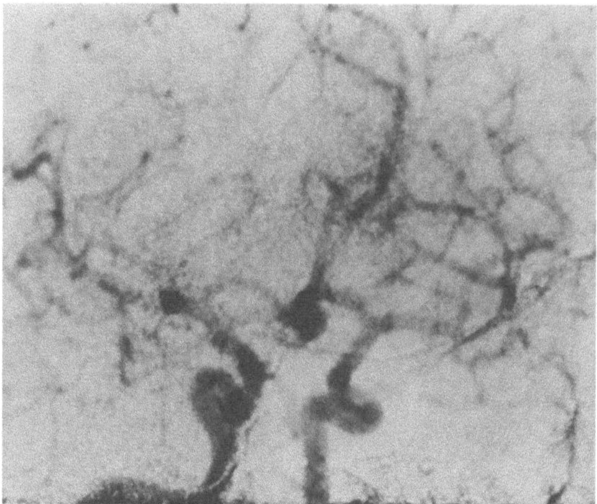

Fig. 7. This is an intracranial study demonstrating an aneurysm at the junction at the left anterior cerebral and anterior communicating arteries

radiographic room we have been successful in reducing all the many types of noise to a minimum.

Figure 5 demonstrates an occlusion of the left subclavian artery with filling of the subclavian via "steal". Figure 6 is an example of an anomalous right subclavian artery and Fig. 7 is an example of an intracerebral study; an aneurysm of the anterior cerebral artery. We have been using more and more of the intravenous studies for intracranial work and are beginning to see detail down to the 1- to 2-mm vessel level.

Abdominal: Fig. 8 represents an intravenous study of severe atherosclerotic involvement of the abdominal aorta. We have been quite successful in using this method in screening hypertensive patients for renal artery stenosis (*Hillman* et al., to be published a) and have concluded that digital video subtraction angiography screening for renovascular hypertension seems medically and economically sound. We have also been quite successful in the evaluation of potential renal donors and renal allograft recipients (*Hillman* et al., to be published b).

Digital subtraction angiography has depicted the number and position of renal arteries preoperatively in renal donors and excluded the presence of renal arterial or parenchymal disease.

It is now the procedure of choice for these referrals in our institution.

Pulmonary: we have had limited experience with pulmonary angiography but are successful when using the technique to define pulmonary emboli in major and middle-sized pulmonary vessels. Figure 9 is an example of a video subtraction angiogram in a dog. We have had comparable visualization in some of our human patients.

Cardiac: Fig. 10 demonstrates an intravenous subtraction video angiogram of the left atrium, left ventricle, and aorta in a dog. Comparable visualization has been defined in humans. Obviously, this must be recorded in real time requiring 30 frames per second. Our original system block diagram shows a Bell and Howell

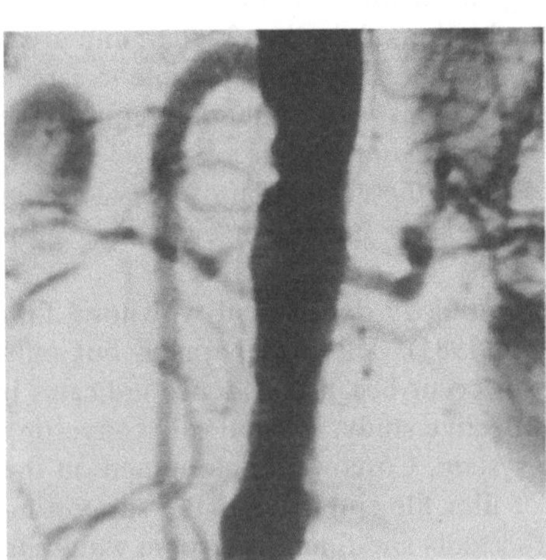 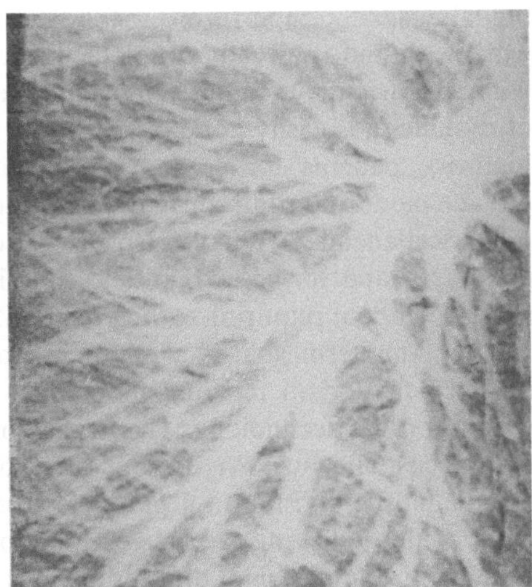

Fig. 8   **Fig. 9**

Fig. 8. This is an intravenous subtraction angiogram demonstrating fairly good detail of the atheromatous changes of the abdominal aorta

Fig. 9. This is an intravenous subtraction pulmonary angiogram demonstrating fairly good detail even of some of the smaller pulmonary arteries. This has been helpful in diagnosing pulmonary emboli in the major and middle-sized vessels

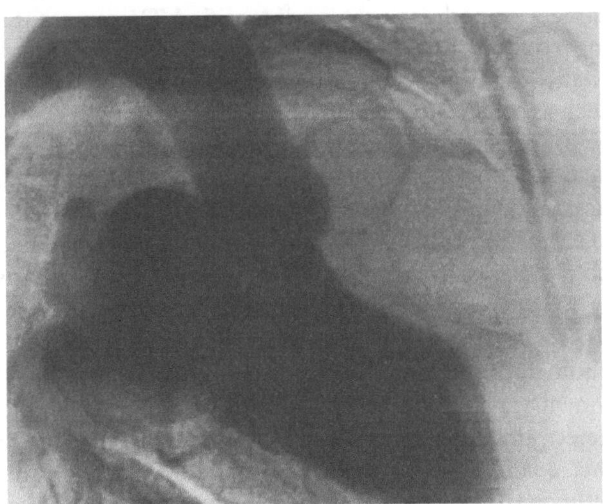

Fig. 10. This is a ventriculogram in a dog demonstrating the left atrium, left ventricle, and the coronary artery coming off anteriorly from the aorta

digital magnetic tape recorder for this function. However, this unit is difficult to work with and is already obsolete. Faster digital recorders that are easier to work with are currently commercially available. Evaluation of ejection fraction and areas of dyskinesia is easily done in real time. Our long-term goal is to be able to screen high-risk patients for coronary artery disease. This will probably require the biplane mode and sophisticated digital tape recording in real time.

Miscellaneous: we have also been successful in the evaluation of the vessels in the upper and lower extremities. This is particularly helpful in evaluating graft patency without requiring catheterization.

Our long-term goal is a photoelectronic radiology department with total film replacement for all imaging modalities (*Capp* 1981). This will happen, but only with improved technology. This transition will occur because evidence indicates it will be cost effective. We did our own cost-effective study, theoretically converting our diagnostic division to a photoelectronic system. Costs were determined on the basis of the following factors: elimination of film file storage and the supporting personnel, elimination of darkroom techs, processors and film. Each room would be equipped with image intensifiers and the entire department and hospital would be automated with storage and retrieval systems. We estimated, on a basis of 65 000 diagnostic examinations per year, that 5 million dollars would be saved over a 10-year period. Extrapolating this to converting all radiology departments in the United States, demonstrates a savings to the health care industry of 1 billion dollars per year. Obviously, many assumptions must be made in this calculation, but the figures are probably on the conservative side. The photoelectronic radiology department of the future will be systems oriented with computers, displays, memory banks, and all the sophisticated technology for both real-time and static imaging. There needs to be much improvement in the detector systems. For example, it is unclear at the present time as to whether the detector receiving the image from the patient will be an image intensifier coupled to optics and TV camera as exists today, or whether it will be an intensifier screen coupled to a TV camera or perhaps even an intensified TV camera. Size has been a limiting factor in receptors except for the intensifier screen (electrodelca lens). Sixteen- and twenty-inch image intensifiers will shortly be available. Other types of detectors, such as solid state, may also be feasible.

In considering photoelectronics as a replacement for film, the real problem lies in evaluating the degradation compared with the diagnostic x-ray film. We did a lung nodule study that showed a 1024 × 1024 TV system to be equal to film (*Seeley* et al. 1978). This was a small limited study conducted by radiologists evaluating both systems. There obviously needs to be an extensive psychophysical evaluation of all the components, including the radiologists.

To test the TV camera degradation alone, seven sets of pediatric cases were photographed from a view box as well as from a 1024 line TV monitor. These were shown via slides to several groups of radiologists who were unable to subjectively detect any difference. We are close to achieving the technical sophistication where the quality of the digitized image is close to that of film. However, where pulmonary structures are concerned, the process involving digitizing images is not ready to be used. Improvements in technology need to be made and more comparative testing carried out. When that is accomplished there will be immediate retrieval of the image from the storage area to offices, clinics, and wards within the hospital and in some cases, outside the hospital. Within 1 s after the radiographic exposure, the technologist would have access to the image within the examination room. Another option would involve all radiographic images in the department going to quality control for evaluation by the radiologist. All radiographic information would be stored on a laser digital disc recorder and from there, using various memory banks, could be transmitted to the reading room, clinics, offices, etc. Doctors in their own offices would at all times have access to the image as well as to the video report from the radiologist. The educational and service functions in the wards and clinics would be served in the same way, eliminating the inefficiency of clinicians coming down from various parts of the hospital in the day or night seeking out films.

References

Capp MP (1981) Radiological imaging – 2000 A. D. Radiology 138:541–550

Christenson PC, Ovitt TW, Fisher HD et al. (1980) Intravenous angiography using digital video subtraction: Intravenous cervicocerebrovascular angiography. Am J Neuroradiol 1:379–386

Hillman BJ, Ovitt TW, Capp MP, Prosnitz EH, Osborne RW, Goldstone J, Zukoski CF, Malone JM (to be published a) The potential impact of digital video subtraction angiography (DVSA) on screening for renovascular hypertension

Hillman BJ, Zukoski CF, Ovitt TW, Ogden DA, Capp MP (to be published b) Digital video subtraction angiography in the evaluation of potential renal donors and renal allograft recipients

Kruger RA, Mistretta CA, Lancaster J et al. (1978) A digital video image processor for real-time X-ray subtraction imaging. Opt Eng 17:652

Kruger RA, Mistretta CA, Houk TL, et al. (1979) Computerized fluoroscopy in real time for noninvasive visualization of the cardiovascular system: Preliminary studies. Radiology 130:49–57

Nudelman S, Fisher D, Frost M, Capp MP, Ovitt T (to be published) A study of photoelectronic – digital radiology (Part I) The photoelectronic – digital radiology department. IEEE

Ovitt TW, Christenson PC, Fisher HD et al. (1980) Intravenous angiography using digital video subtraction: X-Ray imaging system. AJNR 1:387–390

Roehrig H, Frost M, Baker R et al. (1976) High-resolution low-light level video systems for diagnostic radiology. SPIE 78:102

Roehrig H, Nudelman S, Fisher HD, Frost M, Capp MP (1981) Photoelectronic imaging for radiology. IEEE Trans Nucl Sci NS-28:

Seeley GW, Roehrig H, Nudelman S et al. (1978) Psychophysical evaluation of video systems compared to film. J Appl Photo Eng 4:1978

Digital Subtraction Arteriography (DSA)

A. B. Crummy and C. A. Mistretta [1]

1 Introduction

Digital subtraction arteriography (DSA) has recently generated considerable interest in clinical radiology. The reasons for this are multifacetted; however, two considerations have been paramount: The ease and safety of the intravenous injection of contrast agent and the reduced amount of contrast agent necessary for satisfactory study, and the additional information which can be derived when the contrast agent is injected on the arterial side have been major factors.

These techniques have been the outgrowths of research predominantly conducted at the University of Wisconsin and the University of Arizona over the last decade. It is our purpose to discuss the physical aspects of DSA and to present a clinical perspective.

1 Departments of Radiology and Medical Physics, University of Wisconsin, Clinical Science Center, 600 Highland Avenue, Madison, WI 53792/USA

2 Physical Aspects

The digital x-ray systems currently used for nonfilm subtraction angiography may be divided into two principal categories: (1) image-intensified video fluoroscopy, and (2) scanned linear detection systems. The use of energy as well as time subtraction has been investigated for both systems and several types of algorithms have been employed.

The work of *Brody* et al. (1980) has led us to conclude that by trading imaging speed for reduced scatter and potentially more quantitative transmission information, a clinically usable intravenous angiogram using linear detector systems will be obtained. These systems are particularly well suited for static imaging where energy subtraction techniques and imaging selective materials appear promising.

Our work, which began in 1971, has concentrated on image-intensified video fluoroscopy. In the early 1970's, Kelcz from the University of Wisconsin, used image-intensified fluoroscopy for selected iodine imaging using two (*Crummy* et al. 1973) and three K-edge beam techniques (*Kelcz* and *Mistretta* 1977). *Kruger* et al. (1977) and *Riederer* et al. (1981) extended this early analog video subtraction work by using digital video systems. Heavy filtrations and poor transmission of these beams, which had an average energy in the 30–40 kVp range, resulted in very limited transmission statistics. This proved to be the major limitation. Energy subtraction for intravenous angiocardiography was reported by *Houk* et al. (1979) who used a two-filter, constant kVp approach to produce a dynamic motion-immune display. Because of the restricted capacity of the generator available in the laboratory at that time, the technique had to be limited to subjects of 15 cm or less. Thus, this mode is potentially useful in pediatric angiocardiography.

There is currently intense interest in digital subtraction angiography performed with time subtraction studies. A number of commercial systems are available, and the majority of these employ the video fluoroscopy approach with some differences in the method of how the time subtraction algorithms are carried out.

The time subtraction techniques most commonly used are, in concept, very similar to film subtraction angiography which has been employed for decades. The digital technique nevertheless provides greater flexibility in filming rate and image display. In the serial mode the images are generally generated at rates of ½–2 per second. The subtraction mask is taken before the arrival of the contrast agent in the area of interest, and in studies of the thorax this must be prior to the injection. In fluoroscopic mode where a continuous series of subtraction images are generated at normal video rates of 30 frames/second, the mask is obtained prior to the injection because these studies are generally used to evaluate the heart. Recently there have been numerous reports in the literature detailing the use of these modes, as well as a time image difference mode (TID) which shows short-term changes in iodine distribution (*Brennecke* et al. 1977; *Kruger* et al. 1978, 1979a, b; *Meaney* et al. 1980; Ovitt et al. 1978).

2.1 Data Acquisition, Real Time Processing, and Storage

Data acquisition, real time processing, and storage are so interrelated that it is virtually impossible to consider them independently. For example, the type of data storage which can be utilized is dependent upon the extent to which the data has been digitally processed and contrast enhanced before storage. Likewise, the requirements for the video system depend upon the extent to which one wishes to integrate the transmission data over time.

The requirements for the x-ray generator are very much dependent upon the clinical imaging to be undertaken. Important factors are the statistical x-ray transmission requirements which depend upon the spatial resolution desired and the anticipated contrast of the objects to be studied. The exposure time requirements vary with the expected amount of arterial pulsation which results in lateral movement. Thus, examination of the coronary arteries with an intravenous injection of contrast agent, a technique which as yet has no proven clinical applicability, would require an x-ray generator capable of delivering 1000 MA or more in order that exposure times of 10 ms can be achieved. For less demanding clinical applications, longer exposure times may be used in connection with data integration, either on the target of the television camera or in digital memory. In those instances where one would be examining the aorta, peripheral vessels, or carotid arteries, the x-ray generator only needs to deliver currents in the order of 400–500 MA.

The requirements for the x-ray focal spot are similar to those of many other radiographic imaging situations. Aspects to be considered in this context are the focal spot size, the magnification to be used, and the limiting resolution of the digital video system. When a 512×512 pixel matrix covers a 6-inch image intensifier, the degradation of the resolution by a 1-mm focal spot is approximately equal to that provided by the limited pixel matrix at a magnification of about 1.5. However, larger magnifications could be employed without limiting resolution with a 256×256 matrix and the same 1-mm focal spot. For the most part, digital video angiography has been carried out with focal spots of between 0.6 mm and 1.2 mm with magnification factors of 1.5 or less.

We at the University of Wisconsin have not studied the role of x-ray grids for digital video arteriography in any detail and not much has been published in this area. Our original laboratory system had an air gap of 10–15 cm, and it was our impression that the use of grids did not result in striking improvement in image quality in the case of small fields, such as might be used to study the carotid artery in the neck or intracranially. Additional work is needed in this area before a definitive statement can be made.

Generally, the television system, rather than the image intensifier, limits the spatial resolution of this system. Therefore, design of future image intensifiers might emphasize detection efficiency rather than spatial resolution. Two of the more important limitations associated with the image intensifier are limited size and the lateral communication of transmitted intensity information commonly called veiling glare. There has been interest in using larger image intensifiers in order to evaluate larger areas with the limited number of iodine contrast injections which can be used in any diagnostic study. For example, a six- or nine-inch image-intensifier format will not allow adequate simultaneous study of both lungs or kidneys. Therefore, a larger image intensifier might provide a definite advantage. However, the use of the larger intensifier has the inherent disadvantage that scatter increases with field size. In addition, a larger image pixel matrix is required to maintain spatial resolution.

Scatter and glare must be properly accounted for in order to extract quantitative transmission information from image-intensifier systems. It is common that 50% or more of the apparent transmission in a particular picture element is due to effects other than the primary x-ray transmission. Therefore, it is necessary to correct for these effects before the logarithmic processing. Multiple approaches to minimize these problems have been implemented or suggested, for example, the improved contrast ratio of recently introduced large-format image intensifiers, air-gap magnification techniques, and possible use of grids for new multisplit devices.

The requisite performance of the television camera is very dependent upon the circumstances of the clinical imaging situation. Such factors as the signal to noise ratio, spatial resolution, and lag characteristics are important. In the University of Wisconsin laboratory we have used cameras with signal to noise ratios between 200-1 and 1200-1. In the clinical situation, a signal to noise ratio of 2–300:1 seems to provide images which are adequate, especially when image integration is used. However, higher signal to noise ratios ae required in situations with a broad range of transmission values. The relative importance of quantum statistical noise and video noise alters with scene brightness. Generally quantum noise dominates in bright areas while video noise is the primary limitation in dark areas. Thus, in an examination of coronary artery bypass grafts, where one is dealing with an opacified ventricle and aorta as well as the lucent lungs, a high dynamic range television camera is a necessity.

The spatial resolution potential of the television camera is also important. Contrast levels are usually quite low following the intravenous injection of contrast agent, so that a digital matrix size of 512×512 using a six- or nine-inch format is generally a good combination with the x-ray exposure levels employed. However, if one were to use a large-format image intensifier (14-inch) with a pixel matrix of 1024×1024, a camera capable of higher spatial resolution is necessary. In either instance, one can increase the quality of the examination by achieving a higher contrast level. This may be achieved by intra-arterial injection. The combination of the intra-arterial injection with a high spatial resolution television system allows one to approach the quality of film arteriography.

The signal from the television camera may be digitized either before or after the logarithmic processing. However, since the logarithmic amplifier does not appreciably increase the video noise, there is little advantage to digitization after log processing. In instances with especially high contrast signals, the use of a logarithmic look-up table removes the necessity to consider possible limitations of gain bandwidth product. When logarithmic amplification is used to stretch the dark areas of the video scene, 8-bit digitization is generally adequate. When digitization precedes logarithmic processing, the required number of gray levels in the dark portion of the image necessitates the use of 10-bit digitization. An advantage of using a logarithmic look-up table is that first order beam-hardening corrections can be included in the table.

The majority of commercially available systems employ real time digital memory buffers and subtraction so that the fully processed images can be viewed during passage of the contrast bolus through the area of interest. Recording of un-processed data in digital form is an alternative which has a slight advantage in that the technician need not make a selection of the expected contrast ranges. In situations where the real time data is displayed as a subtraction image prior to the display, some choice has to be made with regard to the amount of contrast enhancement to be employed. In practice, there is no reason for not displaying the data in real time, except in the presence of extreme amounts of motion. The possibility exists that if analog data storage is used, the very bright and dark signals may be limited to a predetermined maximum black and white level. This would preclude processing to recover data deteriorated by patient motion. However, the analog levels can usually be set so as to provide a large enhancement factor and a very low incidence of clipping.

Another advantage of the analog relative to digital storage is an economic one. For devices of similar cost, the analog will have a higher storage and frame rate capacity. For the most part, currently commercially available digital subtraction angiographic systems, employing purely digital storage, are limited to one to two frames per second at 512×512 or six to eight frames at 256×256. On the other hand, the analog systems using a 512×512 matrix can function at a rate of 30 reconstituted video signals per second, with very little degradation of the resolution or signal to noise ratio. It must be kept in mind that successful use of analog storage devices requires that the subtraction data must be fully processed and enhanced by digital means. When this is done, the iodine information is enhanced by a large factor relative to that which would be stored prior to subtraction. The digital preprocessing under these circumstances has an effect equivalent to multiplying the signal to noise ratio by the enhancement factor used. When the isolated iodine information is amplified, the quantum statistical fluctuations are similarly amplified. Thus, the noise fluctuations associated with analog recording devices are relatively insignificant, and even after redigitization of the data stored on the analog device, the quantum statistical noise predominates.

A real time digital video recording device, consisting of multiple disc surface connected in parallel so as to produce bit transfer rates of 100 MHz, has recently been constructed in our laboratory. This piece of equipment combines the advantages of the high frame rates presently provided by the analog storage devices with the advantages of digital storage. The system has not been completely evaluated, and whether such a device will be included in commercial systems will largely be dictated by economic factors.

Digital data compression schemes may be used to limit the amount of data to be stored and therefore reduce the cost of the digital storage requirements. Simple subtraction is a step in this direction as far as data compression is concerned. If the more sophisticated data compression schemes which are available can be implemented in real time, their use should be advantageous.

Archival storage of digital subtraction angiography data can be carried out in a number of ways. In clinical practice, the use of a multiformat camera to record the images has proved to be eminently satisfactory. The images are then readily available for the angiographers to interpret and for review by clinicians. Storage of dynamic data had to be carried out with the use of videotape.

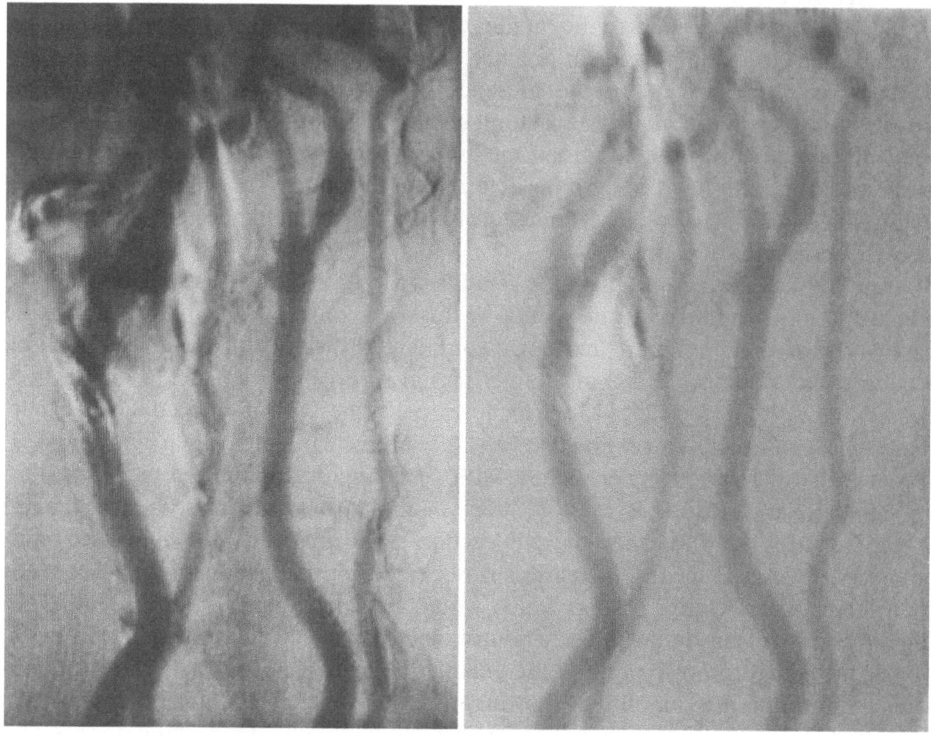

Fig. 1 a, b. Digital subtraction arteriogram of a patient suspected of having transient ischemic attacks. In **a**, the left carotid bifurcation is well delineated and normal. The right carotid bifurcation is not easily seen because the patient swallowed. The movement of air in the pharynx has resulted in a degraded image. Selection of another mask and reprocessing has largely eliminated the artifact so that we can see that the right carotid bifurcation is also normal

2.2 Postprocessing

The greatest limitation seen in clinical digital subtraction arteriography is that of patient motion which occurs between the mask and the time of opacification. When this occurs the video fluoroscopy system has a great advantage over the slit scan system, in that it is possible to obtain a large number of alternate masks during passage of the contrast agent. Following recording of the subtraction images, alternate masks may be used so that one which more closely approximates the position of the patient at the time of opacification can be used (Fig. 1 a, b). Usually this process results in a number of successful registrations in which one can adequately cancel nonvascular anatomy and adequately display the arteriogram. The selection of an alternate mask may be carried out easily using analog as well as digital information, provided that the appropriate enhancement factors have been chosen prior to analog storage. This is not a problem in practice since the degree of opacification for any particular type of examination is relatively predictable. It is important to keep in mind that this remasking procedure does not require the storage of unsubtracted information. The subtraction of pairs of subtracted images cancels the original mask, and produces a new subtraction images in which the first image serves as a mask for the second.

A potential solution to the problem of patient motion is the registration of image pairs through rotation and translation or distortion of one of the images. With the original University of Wisconsin system, we have been able to move images both horizontally and vertically. In rare instances, we were able to obtain relatively spectacular results with this limited reregistration capacity. However, it soon became apparent that the motions of overlying anatomy were far more complicated than that which could generally be restored by simple translation of the images. We are pessimistic that rotation will be sufficient to solve the problem. However, it may be possible to achieve reregistration on a local basis, even if it is not possible over the entire image. The use of more complicated algorithms, involving stretching of the image between recognizable fiducial points provided by bony landmarks, is a possible approach. It must be emphasized that all such algorithms are capable of producing occasional dramatic image restorations. The question remains of how large a fraction of patients will benefit from such image manipulation.

2.3 Quantitative Analysis

The image-intensified fluoroscopy video signal does not directly represent the line integral of the attenuation coefficients of the patient. Superimposed upon this signal is the contribution from x-ray scatter and from the veiling glare. Because of this, we would like to stress that even though the data is digital, it should not be assumed that it is quantitatively accurate. It should not be construed that because the digital data from computerized tomography provided relatively quantitative data, digital subtraction angiography, because it is also digital, will also provide such quantitative data. It may be possible to obtain accurate quantitative data if corrections are made to allow for the signals from the scatter radiation and glare.

These inaccuracies in the uncorrected data do not necessarily preclude them from being useful in certain clinical problems. This is particularly true when the clinical problem involves the measurement of transmission ratios. Also, if one is interested in the time of maximum opacification of an artery, the measurement should be accurate despite the discussed limitations.

Initial work in our laboratory encourages us to believe that it should be possible to devise reliable algorithms, for determining such quantitative functions as cardiac ejection fraction and percent reduction in a lumen of an artery. While most quantitative functions such as cardiac ejection fraction and percent reduction in a lumen of an artery will probably involve the use of digital data to obtain absolute or relative volume estimates of total iodine concentration, less complex calculations based on algorithms such as the area length method may also be employed. *Ludwig* and *Engels* (1981) have utilized the TID mode to calculate cardiac ejection fractions based on area length methods, and have found these to correlate well with calculations based on cineangiography.

Many of the quantitative procedures of nuclear medicine will most likely be investigated using the digital subtraction angiography approach. The DSA approach would have the additional advantage of higher resolution of the anatomic information. Additional statistical limitations associated with the nuclear images could be overcome.

2.4 New Algorithms

It is hoped that new imaging algorithms can be developed to deal with some of the problems which remain in the area of digital subtraction angiography. With the use of the intravenous injection of contrast agent, patient motion is the most severe problem. Preliminary information developed by *Sackett* and *Mann* (1980) at the University of Wisconsin suggests that present algorithms used in conjunction with nonionic contrast material will allow us to be successful in the large majority of clinical studies. Other algorithms will be required to improve our ability to satisfactorily study the coronary arteries and coronary artery bypass grafts.

For nonangiographic application, where iodine has accumulated in organs over a period too long to employ time subtraction, various forms of energy subtraction may be important. One of the major limitations in digital subtraction arteriography is the small field which can be covered by the image intensifier. If it were possible to develop instrumentation which would permit the storage of multiple masks so the entire course of the contrast agent in the lower extremity could be studied with a single injection, the utility of the technique would be markedly enhanced. This would be particularly important in patients such as diabetics in whom limitation of the contrast burden is particularly desirable. It is likely that significant patient motion could be eliminated by the use of nonionic contrast agent, and this, coupled with the relatively low incidence of significant motion in the lower extremities (in the absence of pain), would make it seem that time-dependent subtraction arteriography might be possible using a line scan system. For such an application, a large area of image coverage would be particularly advantageous. Because of the low overall attenuation of the extremities, relatively poor data acquisition rates of such a system would not appear to impose an undue limitation, and the need for alternative masks would likely be less than in other areas of the body such as the abdomen.

Investigation of the heart represents the area in which DSA may be improved the most. In cardiac applications, use of an integrated blurred mask prior to real time subtraction may result in tissue misregistration artifacts which may be mistaken for arterial structures. Using data stored on a disc has convinced us that a cardiac-phased matched subtraction mask will improve the quality of cardiac examinations. However, this is an extremely time-consuming chore. We have used EKG gating to obtain phase-related subtractions at end systole and end diastole but have found dynamic displays to be more beneficial in identifying moving coronary arteries and grafts. Therefore, we are working on a real time display in which a series of EKG-labeled preinjection masks will be subtracted from similarly identified postinjection information in real time. It has been decided to incorporate this algorithm in the semiconductor memory of a new imaging system we are building, rather than utilizing a real time digital disc. Whether this will be cost effective remains to be seen.

At the time that computerized tomography was introduced clinically, it was apparent that considerable improvement could be expected within a short time. However, we do not think that similar improvements can be anticipated as rapidly in digital subtraction angiography. The early CT images were limited by the detector, small matrix sizes, and relatively crude reconstruction algorithms. In DSA, the algorithms are relatively simple, and a method of improving them in any simple manner is not immediately apparent. Furthermore, the image intensifiers and television systems are highly sophisticated because of considerable previous research and application. The major limiting factors in intravenous DSA are the quantum statistics and patient motion. Advances in the image-intensifier tubes and television cameras will not greatly improve upon these problems. Therefore, we do not expect the rapid change in the digital subtraction arteriography which occurred in the field of computerized tomography.

3 Clinical Aspects

3.1 Injection Technique

The enhanced contrast resolution of the digital subtraction technique allows, in many instances, satisfactory opacification of the arterial system following intravenous injection of contrast agent. This of course has considerable appeal because the inherent safety of the intravenous access makes outpatient arteriography feasible. Initially we used hand injections through needles placed in the antecubital fossa. It soon became apparent that this technique did not consistently provide a satisfactory bolus. We then switched to using a # 16 gauge 4″ angiocath in the basilic vein with power injection. The compactness of the bolus was considerably improved with this technique and the quality of the studies improved appreciably. Nevertheless, there were some distinct disadvantages. Reflux of contrast agent into the veins of the forearm and sequestering of contrast agent in the venous reservoir behind the valves occurred regularly. Less regularly, but nevertheless frequently, reflux of contrast agent into the veins of the neck, or an inadvertent Valsalva maneuver by the patient, interfered with the bolus and imaging of the neck arteries. The major disadvantage, however, was the risk of extravasation if one of the peripheral veins burst. This occurred on several occasions, and while no permanent sequellae resulted, the patients had considerable pain for approximately 8 h (*Crummy* et al. 1980).

In order to obviate these difficulties, we have adopted a technique which utilizes the percutaneous placement of a 5.3 or 6 French catheter in the vena cava just peripheral to the right atrium. For the most part, an upper extremity vein is utilized. If the antecubital veins are unsatisfactory, the femoral vein is an alternative, even in outpatients.

An injection rate of between 12 and 28 cc per second is used and the volume varies between 40 and 56 cc. The larger volume is generally employed for the abdominal aorta and peripheral vesels. A contrast agent which contains between 350 and 400 mg of iodine per cc is used.

The mask must be taken prior to the arrival of the contrast agent, and yet be as close temporally to the contrast agent filled frames as possible in order to reduce the effects of patient motion. In the thorax this means that the mask must be obtained prior to the injection. At other sites one delays the mask for a number of seconds based on an estimate of the circulation time.

The abdominal vessels present a particular problem because bowel gas is superimposed. Peristaltic motion will interfere with subtraction and therefore it should be suppressed. This is readily accomplished by injecting 1 mg glucagon intravenously just prior to the study. After the glucagon injection the catheter should be flushed with saline to prevent precipitation of the glucagon by the contrast agent.

3.2 Projections

Generally, the projections utilized are those which are employed for standard arteriography. The major exception to this is in the evaluation of paired vessels, for example, the carotid arteries. In such circumstances use of a standard lateral projection would result in superimposition because of the total opacification of the vascular tree. We have found the use of a Carm image-intensifier mount to be very useful. This obviates the need to move the patient for an oblique projection, but this is achieved instead with angulation of the x-ray apparatus. When the patient is supine and relatively comfortable, the likelihood of patient motion disrupting the examination is reduced. One can also obtain cranial or caudal angulation if this is desirable.

The rate of filming depends of course upon the clinical problem. Generally, film exposures are obtained at one per second for mask mode radiography. However, the apparatus can be programmed to take films as rapidly as two and a half per second. In the continuous mask mode fluoroscopy up to 30 frames per second can be obtained (512×512 format). This is particularly useful in studying the heart and is very useful if one gives intra-arterial injections. Because the image is seen immediately on the television screen, imaging can be terminated as soon as the desired information has been obtained.

3.3 Elements of a Satisfactory Examination

Three elements are essential for a satisfactory examination. First, one must have a cooperative patient. If the patient is unable to remain immobile for any reason, the examination will not be satisfactory. Secondly, because of the decreased contrast available with intravenous injection, inordinately large patients are generally not suitable. Thirdly, the problem must be appropriate. Evaluation of large vessels such as the cervical carotid and the subclavian arteries for stenoses is very well carried out. Similarly, evaluation of postoperative vascular grafts is easily carried out because the vessels and prostheses are generally large and can be well opacified. However, evaluation of the intracranial vasculature for very subtle neoplastic changes with an intravenous injection of contrast agent is not satisfactory, nor is the examination of gastrointestinal bleeders. In the first instance, the spatial resolution is not adequate and in the second hyperperistalsis and overlap will compromise the examination.

3.4 Current Clinical Indications

Based on our experience and that of others, it is clear that digital subtraction arteriography has some utility as a screening test, as an alternative to standard arteriography, and as a technique for obtaining arteriographic information which cannot be obtained with conventional arteriograms, in addition to being a useful aid in the performance of some interventional arteriographic procedures.

3.5 Screening

Heretofore, screening for cervical cerebral vascular disease has been largely restricted to the identification of hemodynamically significant stenoses. The assessment of the possible presence of nonobstructing ulcerative atheroma has not been successful. Digital subtraction arteriography allows one to identify nonobstructing ulcerative plaques as well as stenoses. However, the identification of the ulcers because they may be more subtle, is not as satisfactory as the demonstration of obstruction. This is not surprising when one considers that all ulcerative plaques cannot be identified using standard arteriography (Fig. 1).

Recently, a comparison study of carotid bifurcation arteriography carried out by digital subtraction technique and the conventional technique was reported (*Weinstein* et al. 1980). The DSA examination was bilaterally good to excellent in 60%, and unilaterally good to excellent in an additional 23% of patients. The overall sensitivity of the digital examination was 95% with a specificity of 99% and accuracy of 97%. This experience, and that of others, indicates that digital subtraction arteriography is an excellent means of evaluating patients for the presence of potentially correctable lesions in the cervical carotid arteries.

Screening of patients for renal vascular hypertension has been an area of interest for years. It is widely accepted that the intravenous pyelogram, which has been the cornerstone of case finding, is not very satisfactory. The combination of digital subtraction arteriography with intravenous pyelography results is a worthwhile extension of the urographic examination. Since contrast agent is utilized for both examinations, the digital technique can be carried out without any additional risk. *Hillman* et al. (1980) at the University of Arizona have reported a satisfactory examination rate of 92% with a high degree of diagnostic accuracy, in the evaluation of renal arteries in patients studied with a variety of renal-related clinical indications.

3.6 An Alternative to Standard Arteriography

Digital subtraction arteriography may be used as an alternative to standard studies in a wide variety of vascular problems. Examination of the central pulmonary arteries is very satisfactory and we have been able to demonstrate pulmonary emboli there as well as to distinguish enlarged pulmonary hila from neoplasms. The peripheral pulmonary arteries are not as well evaluated and on occasion we have not been able to demonstrate the presence of emboli which were known to be present on the basis of previous standard examinations (*Crummy* et al. 1980).

The problem is primarily related to the inability of these dyspneic patients to suspend respiration. This means that most patients with pulmonary emboli are not good candidates for evaluation with this technique. An exception to this would be the patient who is on assisted respiration. In these individuals apnea can be induced for the few seconds which are required for the examination.

We have been very satisfied with the evaluation of pulmonary arteriovenous fistulae. We have been able to demonstrate very small fistulae which could not be seen on a plain film. These studies can be conducted with less than 20 cc of contrast agent and are very well tolerated by the patients.

There is considerable interest in the evaluation of left ventricular wall motion by DSA (*Crummy* et al. 1980; *Shaw* et al. 1980). This is done in the time image difference mode and areas of akinesia or dyskinesia which are profiled are readily identified. Areas of the myocardium which are out of phase are seen in anomalous shades of black or white.

The possibility of calculating left ventricular ejection fractions is under active investigation. A major advantage of the technique is that no assumption need be made about ventricular shape. The outline of the ventricle is traced by a light pen and the position of the aortic and mitral valves determined. Then the amount of iodine contained within the boundary is determined.

Two problems are immediately apparent. One is the density which is super-imposed by the pulmonary vasculature and the other is the lack of uniform density of the image-intensifier field. In the first instance, because the amount of contrast in the pulmonary vasculature between systole and diastole will remain relatively constant, it will probably not present a problem. Whether the lack of the uniform density in the image-intensifier field would render the information unsuitable for clinical use has not been determined. However, techniques for eliminating this lack of uniformity have been extensively investigated by Riederer and Shaw in our Department, and solutions to the problem are being pursued.

Because of rapid motion, small size, and frequent subtlety of important changes, evaluation of the coronary arteries has not been clinically useful. We have been able to identify coronary artery bypass grafts, and to this extent the DSA examination of coronary artery disease may be of some utility. However, in the instance of occluded grafts, because the information is negative, one is always faced with the possibility that failure to identify the graft may be related to technical factors rather than due to occlusion. Assessment of both the aortic and coronary anastomoses is not very good and is a leading source of dissatisfaction with this approach.

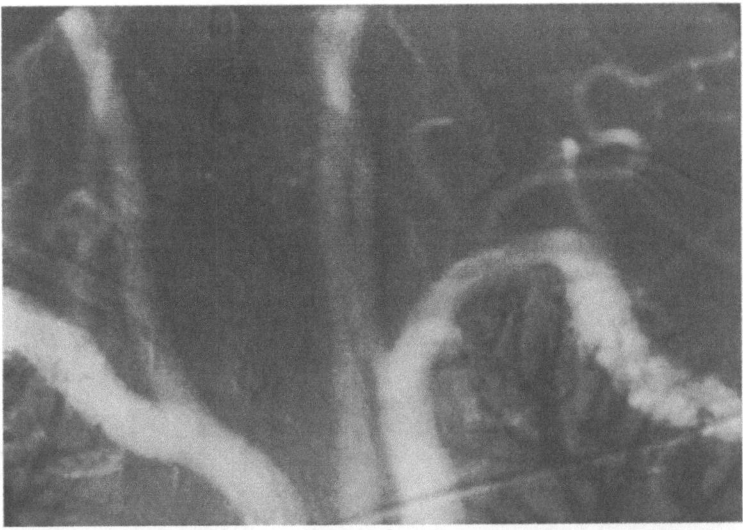

Fig. 2. A 28-year-old female was seen because of intermittent numbness in the left upper extremity which was felt to be related to the thoracic outlet syndrome. Physical examination showed diminution of pulse in Adson's position. In addition, there was a mass palpable in the left supraclavicular fossa. The possibility that this represented an aneurysm was entertained. Digital subtraction arteriography carried out with the intravenous injection of 56 cc of contrast agent shows that the left subclavian artery is somewhat elongated and extends more superiorly than is usual. No evidence of an aneurysm is seen

The thoracic aorta and brachiocephalic vessels are ideal for evaluation by intravenous digital subtraction arteriography. Because of the aorta's large size, dense opacification is readily achieved. We have been very satisfied with our ability to delineate anomalies and aneurysms as well as athero-ulcerative disease. The distinction of aneurysms from juxta-aortic neoplasms is readily carried out and has proved to be of considerable clinical utility. Our experience with dissecting hematomas is limited to one case and in this instance, even though we knew that the lesion was present, we were unable to identify the intimal flap. This was very early in our experience and our techniques, as well as the quality of the images, have improved considerably, so that this limited negative experience should not be used to preclude further investigation in this area.

Our experience with brachiocephalic arteriography has been extremely good. The ready demonstration of the subclavian arteries makes patients suspected of thoracic outlet syndrome ideal candidates (Fig. 2). Subclavian and innominate obstructions and stenoses are easily delineated.

Without any question the area of greatest interest and application thus far in intravenous digital subtraction arteriography has been the evaluation of patients with cervical carotid artery disease. In many instances the quality of screening digital subtraction carotid or vertebral arteriograms is sufficient for preoperative decisions, and a standard arteriogram may be omitted.

The abdominal aorta has also been a fruitful area for investigation by digital subtraction arteriography. The relationships between abdominal aortic aneurysms

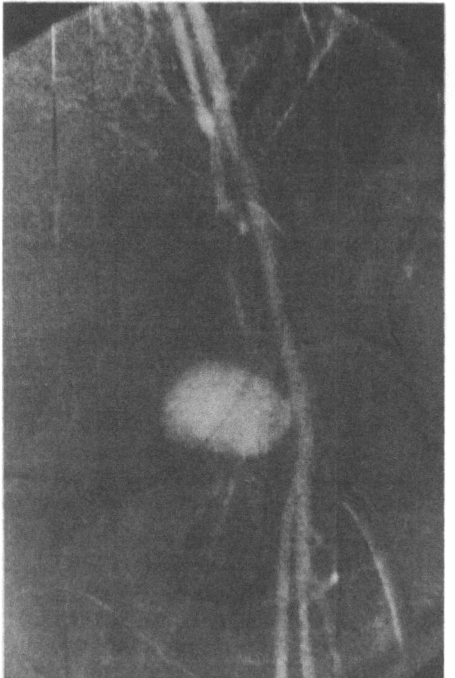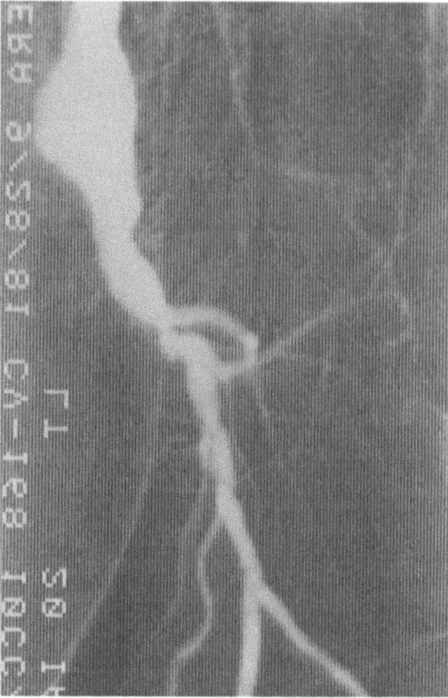

Fig. 3   **Fig. 4**

Fig. 3. This patient had undergone left transfemoral arterial catheterization. Subsequently, she became hypotensive and developed tachypnea and tachycardia. There was no evidence of a hematoma in her groin; however, a radiograph of the abdomen suggests a retroperitoneal hematoma. The DSA performed with the intravenous injection of 50 cc of contrast agent showed a false aneurysm arising from the left common femoral artery and extending through the femoral canal into the retroperitoneal space. This study allowed the surgeons to make an extra-abdominal incision to control the hemorrhage rather than one in the flank

Fig. 4. A 15 cc injection into the abdominal aorta outlines the distal anastomosis of an aorto bifemoral graft. In addition, it shows that the superficial femoral artery is obstructed and that the profunda femoral artery has a high-grade obstruction just distal to the take off of the lateral femoral circumflex. There are also several areas of less severe narrowing distal to this

and the renal arteries, and the possible presence of supernumerary renal arteries is readily determined with DSA and standard studies are obviated. The examination does not provide sufficient detail to examine the peripheral visceral vessels with an intravenous examination.

Digital subtraction arteriography has wide application as an alternative to standard arteriography in the pre- and postoperative assessment in patients with peripheral vascular disease (*Crummy* et al., to be published). The demonstration of infrarenal aortic obstruction, and then of the vessels just distal to the inguinal ligament, is easily done, and provides all the information necessary for preoperative planning for an aortal bifemoral bypass. Postoperatively, one can easily assess juxtaprothetic masses to assess whether they are pseudoaneurysms or other problems. Patency of grafts is readily determined, as well as the state of anastomoses.

Many of the extremity vessels are easily seen. We have been very satisfied with the delineation sites of bleeding with pseudoaneurysm formation following catheterization or other trauma (Fig. 3). One can readily demonstrate whether a large vessel was traumatized by a penetrating injury.

Evaluation of patients with atherosclerotic peripheral vascular disease frequently requires that the abdominal aorta, pelvic, and bilateral extremity vessels be studied. Because the size of the DSA field is limited by the size of the image intensifier one cannot at any one session make a sufficient number of injections to study this large area. Therefore, routine use in peripheral vascular disease is not advocated. Nevertheless, if the clinical circumstances are such that one knows the area of interest, then the digital subtraction approach is quite useful.

3.7 Additional Information Related to Improved Contrast Resolution

The improved contrast resolution of the digital subtraction technique should allow one to identify concentration of contrast agents with DSA which cannot be identified with film. This is true with the intravenous technique but more commonly with arterial injections.

For example, we have been able to identify the cavernous portion of a carotid artery which was completely occluded in the neck, following injection of an intravenous bolus when we could not identify this with selective carotid arteriography. Two factors came into play: (1) the improved contrast resolution of the digital technique; (2) flow in all of the collateral vessels delivered contrast to the area.

The improved resolution may be useful following intra-arterial injection. The widest application of this is in the examination of peripheral vessels distal to severe obstructions. We perform arteriography routinely under these circumstances following the induction of reactive hyperemia. This is accomplished by inflating a blood pressure cuff to above systolic pressure for 7 min. Following deflation, the reative hyperemia invariably results in improvement of flow into the distal regions. However, arteriograms carried out on the operating table with direct injection into the distal vessels have shown that one cannot confidently exclude patent arteries, because of failure to be identified with the standard arteriogram. Currently, we are repeating the arterial injection in a similar manner with the recording being done by the digital subtraction technique. On a number of occasions, we have been able, with DSA, to identify vessels which were satisfactory for bypass but not seen with film recording.

In these circumstances, in two patients who had no runoff identified both proved to be unsatisfactory for bypass. Of the ten patients found to have potentially bypassable vessels, seven were patent with relatively short-term follow up extending from 2 weeks to 15 months. Three early failures have occurred.

We have also utilized this approach for evaluation of patients who have had arteriography performed elsewhere, and who on the basis of failure to opacify distal vessels were judged to be candidates for amputation. In two such patients we have been able to demonstrate bypassable vessels. Amputation was avoided and their bypasses are patent, albeit with short-term follow-up.

Many patients with vascular disease have compromised renal function and may react adversely to large volumes of contrast agent. Digital subtraction arteriography in conjunction with intra-arterial injections allows the vascular examination to be performed with a great reduction in the contrast burden without sacrifice of diagnostic information. In this selected group of patients, this represents a distinct advantage.

3.8 An Aid in the Performance of Interventional Procedures

One of the major handicaps in performing transluminal therapeutic procedures is to see that the catheter and therapeutic device are in the proper position. Repeat injections of contrast agents after assessing the catheter position may require extemely large volumes and, on occasion are precluded by the fact that the catheter lumen is occupied by the device. This problem is obviated by the use of the digital subtraction technique.

Just prior to the therapeutic intervention one can opacify the artery of interest and freeze the image so that it can be continuously displayed on the TV screen. Then the catheter can be advanced through the image of the area of interest. One can readily recognize if a balloon catheter is passed into the external rather than the internal carotid artery, or whether the transluminal dilatation catheter is in the area of stenosis. Matching the length and diameter of the balloon to the internal lumen of the artery is demonstrated by the previously performed arteriogram. In addition, one can readily recognize the relationship of the catheter tip to any branch vessels and to the aorta. This may avoid embolization of particles to areas which should be avoided.

While our experience with this technique is somewhat limited, it has been very positive and we are extremely enthusiastic and feel that this will become one of the major areas of application.

3.9 Cost Benefit Evaluation

Clearly, if a digital subtraction arteriogram is carried out as an alternative to a standard arteriogram, one can expect considerable reduction in cost. This is particularly true if the examination is carried out on an outpatient rather than on an inpatient basis. Another saving is reduction in the use of film. Because the initial recording is carried out on a video disc or videotape which can be reused following permanent recording of selected images, the amount of film required is markedly reduced. A biplane examination of the abdominal aorta which might require 20 films can be recorded on two films, each of which contains four smaller images. Therefore, the cost of film would be less than one-tenth of standard arteriography and there would be a commensurate saving in storage costs, film chemistry, etc.

In addition, one must consider that the largest use of silver in the world is in the manufacture of x-ray films, and since this is a nonrenewable resource conservation is essential.

Cost saving related to screening is somewhat difficult to document. A prospective study would be necessary to determine the cost effectiveness of screening patients with conditions such as cervical carotid artery disease and hypertension. However, when one considers the economic as well as the social costs and the personal devastation which may result from a stroke, prevention is unquestionably desirable. Widespread screening of patients for cervical cerebral vascular disease with catheter arteriography is not feasible, but use of digital subtraction arteriography with selected outptients for this purpose could prove to be very worthwhile.

The application of DSA to peripheral arteriography, in which preliminary data suggest that it may be possible to place bypass grafts and maintain patency in individuals who in general were heretofore considered candidates for amputation, would be a very positive benefit.

3.10 Practical Problems

The greatest single problem in digital subtraction arteriography is that of patient motion. Much of the motion is the result of the feeling of intense heat and the metallic taste the patient experiences as the contrast agent passes through the vascular tree. To a large extent this problem can be eliminated by the use of nonionic contrast agents. Preliminary data of a double-blind study reported by *Sackett* and *Mann* (1980) associates from the University of Wisconsin has shown the nonionic agents to be superior to the currently employed ionic agents. The major problem rests with the considerable cost of the nonionic agents. It is anticipated that with the great interest of the pharmaceutical industry in this area some less expensive agent will be synthesized, and that in combination with large volume requirements the costs may be reduced.

A major problem with standard arteriography has been the transient or permanent loss of renal function in individuals who have had compromised renal function, particularly diabetics, at the time of arteriography. The volume of contrast agent required for a standard intra-arterial study recorded with the digital subtraction technique is considerably reduced. Therefore, because the problem is volume related, arteriography in these individuals should be rendered much safer.

3.11 The Future

Our initial clinical experience, now of about 2 years, suggests that the application of digital arteriography, performed both with the intravenous and intra-arterial injections, will continue to increase in the near future. It is our anticipation that considerably more screening will be carried out with the intravenous injections, and that many standard arteriograms will be supplanted by this. In addition, when standard arteriograms are deemed desirable, much of the recording will be carried out with the digital format. It is our expectation that improvement in patient care will result, and that there will be a marked reduction in the cost of arteriography, notwithstanding the initial start-up costs of the digital devices.

References

Brennecke R, Brown TK, Bursch J, Heintzen DH (1977) Computerized videoimage processing with application to cardioangiographic roentgen image series. In: Nagel HH (ed) Digital image processing. Springer, Berlin Heidelberg New York p 244

Brody WR, Macovski A et al. (1980) Intravenous angiography using scanned projection radiography: preliminary investigation of a new method. Invest Radiol 1:220–223

Crummy AB, Mistretta CA, Ort MG, Kelcz F, Cameron JR, Siedband MP (1973) Absorption edge fluoroscopy using quasi-monoenergetic x-ray beams. Invest Radiol 8:402

Crummy AB, Strother CM, Sackett JF (1980) Computerized fluoroscopy: digital subtraction for intravenous angiocardiography and arteriography. AJR 135:1131–1140

Crummy AB, Strother CM, Lieberman RP et al. (1981) Digital video subtraction angiography for evaluation of peripheral vascular disease. Radiology. 141: 33–37

Hillman BJ, Ovitt TW, Nudelman S et al. (1980) Diagnosis of renovascular disease by computerized video subtraction intravenous angiography. 66th Annual Radiological Society of North America Meeting, Dallas, Texas, 1980

Houk TL, Kruger RA, Mistretta CA, Riederer SJ, Shaw CG, Lancaster JC (1979) Real-time digital K-edge subtraction fluoroscopy. Invest Radiol 14:270–278

Kelcz F, Mistretta CA (1976) Absorption edge fluoroscopy using a 3-spectrum technique. Med Phys 3: 159–168

Kruger RA, Mistretta CA, Crummy AB, Sackett JF, Riederer SJ, Houk TL, Goodsitt MM, Shaw CG, Flemming D (1977) Digital K-edge subtraction radiography. Radiology 125:243–245

Kruger RA, Mistretta CA, Lancaster JC, Houk TL, Goodsitt MM, Riederer SJ, Hicks J, Sackett JF, Crummy AB, Flemming D (1978) A digital video image processor for real-time subtraction imaging. Opt Eng 17:652–657

Kruger RA, Mistretta CA et al. (1979a) Computerized fluoroscopy techniques for noninvasive imaging of the cardiovascular system. Radiology 130:49–57

Kruger RA, Mistretta CA, Riederer SJ, Ergun D, Shaw CG, Row GG (1979b) Computerized fluoroscopy techniques for noninvasive study of cardiac dynamics. Invest Radiol 14: 279–287

Ludwig JW, Engels PHC (1981) Digital vascular imaging (DVI). Medicamundi 26/2:68–80

Meaney TF, Weinstein MA, Buonocore E, Pavlicek W, Borkowski GP, Gallagher JH, Suffa B, MacIntrye WJ (1980) Digital subtraction angiography of the human cardiovascular system. SPIE 233:272–278

Ovitt TW, Capp MP, Fisher HD et al. (1978) The development of a digital video subtraction system for intravenous angiography. In: Miller HA, Schmidt EV, Harrison PC (eds) Non-invasive cardiovascular measurements, vol 167. Society of Photo-Optical Instrumentation Engineers, Bellingham Washington, pp 61–65

Riederer SJ, Kruger RA, Mistretta CA, Ergun DL, Shaw CG (1981) Three beam K-edge imaging of iodine using differences between video fluoroscopic images: Experimental results. Med Phys 8/4:480–488

Sackett JF, Mann FA (1980) Contrast media for computerized fluoroscopy. Presented at the Radiological Society of North America Meeting, Dallas, November, 1980

Shaw CG, Crummy AB, Myerowitz PD et al. (1980) Intravenous techniques for cardiac imaging using computerized fluoroscopy. 66th Annual Radiological Society of North America Meeting, Dallas, Texas, 1980

Weinstein MA, Chilcote WA, Modic MT, et al. (1980) Digital subtraction carotid angiography: a comparative study with conventional angiography in 100 patients. 66th Annual Radiological Society of North America Meeting, Dallas, Texas, 1980

Digital Subtraction Angiography: Cleveland Clinic Experience

T. F. Meaney, M. A. Weinstein, E. Buonocore and J. H. Gallagher[1]

1 Introduction

Digital subtraction angiography has provided a method for noninvasive imaging of the cardiovascular system. The method was introduced into clinical practice by several groups of investigators over the last 3 years (*Brennecke* et al. 1977; *Ergun* et al. 1979; *Kruger* et al. 1979 a, b; *Ovitt* et al. 1978, 1979, 1980) and numerous reports quickly appeared attesting to the general interest in the potential of the technique (*Buonocore* et al. 1981; *Chilcote* et al. 1981; *Christenson* et al. 1980; *Crummy* et al. 1980; *Hillman* et al. 1981; *Meaney* et al. 1980 a, b; *Modic* et al. to be published; *Strother* et al. 1980). Because of the simplicity of an intravenous bolus injection of contrast material, examinations can be performed safely on an outpatient basis and at considerable reduction in expense as compared with conventional angiography. The computer-reconstructed images as a result of digitization of the output signal of an image intensifier/television system form the basis of the method. The present success of DSA in producing useful clinical images is due in large part to the improved efficiency of current image intensifier/television systems, and advances in digital image processing, which permit real-time subtraction imaging and virtually instantaneous remasking of the images. The contrast sensitivity of the system allows identification of small concentrations of intra-

---

1 Division of Radiology, The Cleveland Clinic Foundation, 9500 Euclid Avenue, Cleveland, OH 44106/USA

Table 1. Spatial and contrast resolution in radiological imaging techniques

	Spatial resolution line pairs per mm	Threshold contrast for detection of 1-mm objects
Conventional radiography	5	3%
Fluoroscopy	1.2	5%
CT	1	1%
DSA	2	1%

venously injected iodinated contrast materials. Visualization of 1-mm objects at 1% contrast can be achieved with this method.

Conventional film techniques for angiography have been proven to have superior spatial resolution as compared with current digital imaging techniques, but x-ray film suffers in that, at low contrast levels, spatial resolution is inferior to that of DSA. A comparison of spatial and contrast resolution of several radiologic imaging techniques is shown in Table 1.

2 Materials and Methods

One thousand and seven hundred patients were examined with digital subtraction angiography at the Cleveland Clinic Foundation between March 1980 and April 1981. Of these examinations, 71% were for the extracranial carotid circulation, 9% for intracranial angiography, 12% for renal angiography, and 8% for cardiac and peripheral studies.

In the first 100 patients studied, a 2-inch (5 cm) 16- or 18-gauge catheter was inserted into an arm vein for the injection of contrast material. Because of extravasation of contrast material into the arm of each of three patients producing severe pain but no other sequelae, the technique was altered using an 8-inch (20 cm) 16-gauge intracatheter[1] into a brachial arm vein. A small test injection of approximately 2 cc of contrast material is fluoroscopically observed prior to the bolus injection, to insure that the catheter tip is in a vein at least as large in caliber as the catheter, and that there are no sharp angulations in the vein between the catheter tip and the subclavian vein. If, as a result of the test injection, the vein is deemed to be too small or too tortuous, the catheter is repositioned into a larger vein of the ipsilateral or contralateral arm. Using the 20-cm intracatheter, there has been one extravasation of contrast material in the last 1000 cases. Contrast material is injected at the rate of 12–20 cc per second, depending on the size of the arm vein. Forty cc of contrast material (Renografin-76)[2] are injected followed by a flush injection of 25 cc of 5% dextrose and water. For intracranial studies, the volume of contrast material is increased to 50 cc.

---

1 Deseret Intracath, 16-gauge catheter with a 14-gauge needle; Deseret Co., Sandy, Utah 84070, cat. no. 3112
2 E. R. Squibb & Sons, Inc.

Depending on the patient's weight, age, and renal function, up to five injections have been made during a single examination and without sequelae.

Between March 1980 and January 1981, 700 patients were examined on a specially designed research unit. Between January and June of 1981, 1000 patients were examined on a preproduction DSA unit. This later unit utilizes an x-ray tube with a nominal focal spot of 0.6/1.2 mm and a heat capacity of 400 000 heat units. X-rays are produced using a generator of 1000 Ma, and exposure times per frame range from 5–40 ms. X-rays are detected using a trimodal (9-, 6-, 4.5-inch) cesium iodide image-intensifier tube having a resolution of 2–2.5 line pairs per mm. Whenever possible, the smallest image-intensifier mode is used to reduce Compton scatter and to most efficiently utilize the matrix to produce the smallest pixel size.

The television camera consists of a 525-line, specially designed Vidicon camera with a lead oxide tube having a signal-to-noise ratio of approximately 1000 : 1. The video signal is switch selectable for either linear or logarithmic amplification. In virtually all instances logarithmic amplification is utilized.

The signal is digitized using an 8-bit, 30-MHz, analog-to-digital converter with a 30-frame per second capacity at a 512×512 matrix.

A digitized mask image is stored in one of two memories with a capacity of $512 \times 512 \times 12$ bits; and subsequent images containing contrast material, also digitized, are placed in the second memory and subtracted in real time from the mask image. The resultant subtracted images are stored on digital disc. This digitized information is utilized for remasking procedures and derivation of functional data. Only rarely is the original mask the optimum for subtraction. Usually a mask is chosen which is temporally closest to the arrival of contrast material in the region of interest. Often, however, a late mask after clearance of the contrast material, proves most satisfactory in the subtraction process. Stored digital data is also available for functional imaging procedures.

Three matrix sizes are available. The 512×512 matrix is utilized for framing rates up to one per second, 256×256 for up to six frames per second, and 128×128 is available for framing rates up to twelve frames per second. The digital disc storage capacity is related to the matrix size. We are presently using a 160 megabite disc. The stored digital data is archived to magnetic tape for later recall. In addition, a multiformat camera is utilized for hard copy images.

3 Clinical Applications

The clinical applications for digital subtraction angiography by intravenous injection of contrast material are outlined in Table 2. As noted previously, the primary area of application has been in the study of the extracranial carotid circulation at our institution. Depending on the type of institution, the frequency of examinations of various parts of the body will obviously vary.

3.1 Head and Neck

The usual indication for DSA in this group of patients is the history of transient ischemic attacks (TIA's), amaurosis fugax, completed stroke, and signs and symp-

Table 2. Clinical applications of digital subtraction angiography

I. Head & Neck
  1. Carotid arteries
  2. Intracranial
    a. Vascular abnormalities
    b. Neoplasia
 	
II. Chest
  1. Mediastinal masses
    a. Vascular masses
    b. Aortic aneurysms
      1) Arterioscleritic
      2) Dissecting aneurysms
      3) Traumatic aneurysms
  2. Pulmonary arteriography
  3. Parenchymal abnormalities
    a. A-V fistulas
    b. Pulmonary sequestration
	III. Cardiac
	  1. Left ventricular function
	  2. Congenital disease
	  3. Bypass grafts
	
	IV. Abdomen
	  1. Aorta
	  2. Renal arteries
	  3. Mesenteric vessels
	  4. Organs and neoplasia
	  5. Bypass grafts
	
	V. Peripheral
	  1. Vascular occlusion
	  2. Evaluation of grafts

toms of insufficiency of the posterior cerebral circulation. In addition, patients are also studied who have positive direct or indirect studies of the carotid arteries and asymptomatic bruits.

After initial investigations using various degrees of obliquity, we have determined that 70° RPO and LPO projections show the separate origins of the internal and external carotid arteries most frequently and without overlap of the vertebral arteries. Studies are carried out initially with the two oblique views, and then additional injections are made in other oblique projections until the separate origins of the internal and external carotid arteries are identified without overlap. Accurate positioning permits the bifurcations to be included within the 4.5-inch (11.25 cm) image-intensifier field. The advantage of the small intensifier field is that there is less light scatter than with larger image-intensifier fields, and hence an improvement in the perceived density of the contrast within vessels. When contrast limitation is not a problem we obtain an additional 30°, slightly off-lateral view of the carotid siphons for visualization of stenotic or occlusive disease of the intra-cranial arteries.

The usual cause of an unsatisfactory study is misregistration artifacts caused by patients swallowing between acquisition of the mask image and the contrast-containing image. Various methods have been tried to reduce the incidence of the patient swallowing during the examination, such as having the patient inhale through a straw, exhale through a straw, bite their tongue, bite on an external object, and by cooling of the contrast material. We have concluded that none of these maneuvers appreciably assists in reducing the frequency of the swallowing artifact and now no longer mention to the patient that they should not swallow.

Various abnormalities have been examined including partial and complete artherosclerosis obliterans, fibromuscular disease, and intimal ulcerative disease.

Comparative studies of digital subtraction angiography with traditional carotid angiograms were carried out with 100 patients consecutively to evaluate the accuracy of the DSA examination (*Chilcote* et al. 1981). The DSA examinations were rated as good or excellent in quality if the separate origins of the internal and external carotid arteries were well visualized without overlap or superimposition and when the arterial contrast density was good to excellent. It is significant that in only 1 of the 100 patients was there a poor quality DSA examination due to insufficient contrast density in the carotid arteries. It is because of this initial and continuing experience that we believe that placing a catheter in the superior vena cava or the right atrium is unnecessary to provide an adequate concentration of contrast material. In the initial comparative study, the quality of the DSA examination was considered good to excellent in 70% of the patients. Our current experience, using modifications of the technique and additional projections when necessary, has resulted in good visualization of the carotid bifurcations in 85% of patients. A major factor which has contributed to this improvement in the quality of the study is additional injections. Also, in the initial study, if an arm vein could not be catheterized, the study was considered unsuccessful. Presently, if an arm vein cannot be catheterized, which occurs in approximately 1% of the patients, the study is performed with a catheter placed in the inferior or superior vena cava, either by the brachial or, more commonly, the femoral percutaneous route. Also, in our initial study, venous reflux occurred in 1–2% of the patients, producing unsatisfactory images of the arterial circulation. This is usually due either to patients performing a Valsalva maneuver during the injection or because of compression of the superior vena cava by a mediastinal mass. At present, if such a study is inadequate because of venous reflux, it is repeated on the following day after placing of a central catheter.

In evaluating the comparative study, the DSA was interpreted as being correct if it agreed with the conventional angiogram within a range of approximately 10%–20%. In those patients where the carotid bifurcations were well visualized, there was excellent correlation with the conventional angiogram, with a sensitivity of 95%, specificity of 99%, and accuracy of 97%. Conversely, when the bifurcations were not well visualized with DSA, there was a substantial possibility of misinterpretation of the study, and the sensitivity fell to 54%, specificity 70%, and accuracy 64%. A very important asset of digital subtraction angiography over indirect methods of assessment (carotid compression tomography, ultrasound) is that it is immediately obvious when the DSA examination is of good or poor quality and when the bifurcations are not well visualized.

In the comparative study, four ulcerations of the internal carotid artery were visualized by conventional angiography, and all were detected by DSA when the studies were of excellent quality. There were four additional ulcerations in patients who had poor quality DSA, and none was identified. These results indicate the importance of not attempting to make a firm diagnosis when the quality of the DSA study is suboptimum.

Indications for study of the intracranial cerebral circulation have included tumors, fistulas, arteriovenous malformations, aneurysms, and evaluation of patients preoperatively and postoperatively who have undergone intracranial arterial bypass surgery. Filling of the entire intracerebral circulation within the brain is a disadvantage compared to the intravenous administration of contrast material, but specialized views of the area of interest can alleviate most of these problems. Projections which have been used include Waters, basal, and off-lateral projections. In order to improve the quality of the examination within the head, the 512×512 matrix is used in conjunction with the smallest image-intensifier field consistent with the area to be examined.

Comparative studies have also been carried out in 55 patients studied by DSA who also had traditional selective catheter angiography (*Modic* et al., to be published). These studies have shown that two-thirds of the DSA examinations provided as much information as the traditional angiograms, 22% were only partially diagnostic, and 13% nondiagnostic. DSA has now replaced conventional angiography by evaluation of the juxtasellar carotid arteries prior to transphenoidal hypophysectomy.

As noted previously, the simultaneous bilateral filling of arteries can be a disadvantage but, on the venous side, represents an advantage, since flow defects from unopacified blood coming from the other side does not occur. In the study of arteriovenous malformations, while DSA is usually diagnostic, it does not clearly identify the major feeding vessels and has not replaced angiography in preoperative evaluation of patients. However, it has been most useful in the postoperative evaluation to determine the surgical success in the immediate postoperative period.

While large intracranial cerebral aneurysms can easily be identified by DSA, we do not believe that it is adequate to identify small aneurysms. DSA has also been used to determine if hemifacial spasm in a patient is due to a dolichoectatic vessel adjacent to the facial nerve.

3.2 Mediastinum

The usual indication for DSA in the mediastinum has been the evaluation of mediastinal masses where the differential diagnosis includes the possibility of aneurysm and vascular tortuosity (*Meaney* et al. 1980b). The wide variability of contour of the thoracic aorta and brachiocephalic arteries, especially in the older age group, often requires differential diagnosis from solid masses. Traumatic and dissecting aortic aneurysms may present as chest masses with a wide variety of unusual configurations. They may extend either to the right or left of the mediastinum, as well as being located in either anterior or posterior portions. These unusual configurations often present a diagnostic dilemma which is readily soluble with digital subtraction angiography. Moreover, unusual configurations of the main pulmonary arteries and veins requiring differentiation from solid hilar masses represent an additional application of DSA.

3.3 Pulmonary Embolic Disease

While the main pulmonary artery and primary and secondary branches are usually well identified using DSA, consistent visualization of more distal branches of the pulmonary arteries have been disappointing. The nonselective injection of contrast material and the inability of critically ill patients to suspend respiration are major problems. At present, there is no comparative study available for the accuracy of diagnosis of intravenous digital subtraction angiography with conventional angiography in patients with pulmonary emboli.

3.4 Cardiac

In studies carried out so far, DSA of the heart has been used primarily for the study of left ventricular dynamics. Calculation of ejection fraction by DSA in the evaluation of wall motion have been compared with results obtained from conventional angiography. To date, the results have shown a good correlation of the two methods. The technique which we have used consists of framing rates of six per second with short exposure times per frame (5–15 ms), often combined with EKG gating. Postprocessing algorithms are readily applied to the stored digital information for calculation of volume changes in the ventricular chambers and for identification of wall motion defects.

An evaluation of congenital heart disease by DSA is in progress. Framing rates of six per second with a 256×256 matrix permit the course of contrast material through cardiac chambers to be readily identified. The presence of recirculation through septal defects has been identified by cursor placement over the right atrium in six patients. Moreover, complicated congenital derangements of the heart such as single left ventricle, double chambered hearts, anomalous pulmonary venous return, etc. have been diagnosed by DSA and with similar information content as obtained by cardiac catheterization and biplane cineangiography. An obvious disadvantage in the study of congenital heart disease by the intravenous injection technique is that intracardiac pressures and oxygen sampling cannot be obtained.

Visualization of the coronary arteries by intravenous injection remains an unsolved problem. Major portions of both coronary arteries are obscured because of contrast material filling the left ventricle or left atrium at the time of coronary artery filling. However, supra-aortic valvular catheter injections of contrast material, with either EKG gating or nongated exposures, have provided clinically satisfactory images of the entire coronary circulation in a small number of patients. The obvious benefit of such a study is that less technical skill is required with supra-aortic injections and, hence, patient safety is enhanced.

Coronary artery bypass grafts have also been successfully studied using intravenous digital subtraction angiography. The patency of the grafts were established, but the distal runoff into the native coronary circulation could not be identified in any of these patients due to superimposition of the coronaries and contrast-filled cardiac chambers.

3.5 Abdominal and Peripheral

The usual indications for DSA in the abdomen have been for the aorta and the renal arteries. The usual subjects for study are patients for evaluation of arterial hypertension (Fig. 1), occlusive renal artery disease associated with deteriorating renal function, and postoperative evaluation of renal artery bypass grafts and follow-up of patients who have undergone percutaneous transluminal angioplasty. An infrequent indication has been for the diagnosis of renal masses. Patients with suspected renal masses often have suboptimal visualization because of overlying intestinal gas which moves during the examination, despite the administration of glucagon, and produces serious misregistration artifacts.

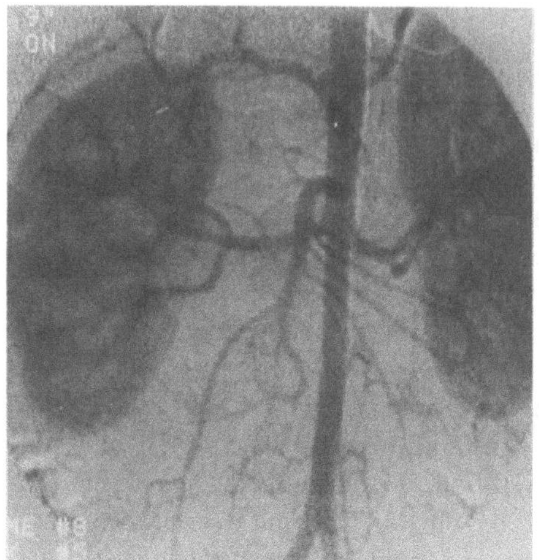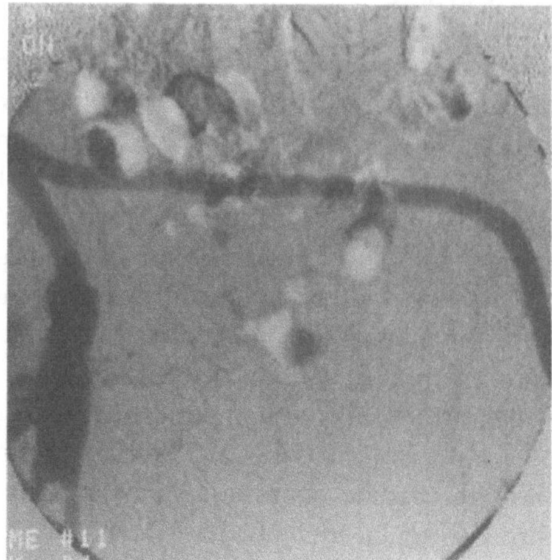

Fig. 1   **Fig. 2**

Fig. 1. Digital Subtraction angiogram of the abdominal aorta in a patient with arterial hypertension showing no evidence of renal artery occlusive disease

Fig. 2. DSA of femoral bypass graft after the peripheral injection of 40 cc of contrast material

During the preliminary experience using the experimental unit, 30 patients were evaluated who had both DSA and conventional catheter abdominal angiography (*Buonocore* et al. 1981). Comparison of the two techniques in this study indicated that 59 of the 70 renal arteries examined were considered to be diagnostic and 11 inadequately visualized. Inadequate visualization was most commonly due to overlying extrarenal arteries. In the 59 arteries that were adequately identified, the findings agreed with the results of traditional selective catheter renal angiography in 50 patients. Five of the patients were overdiagnosed by digital subtraction angiography; that is, a greater degree of stenosis than was found on the conventional angiogram was reported, while four patients were underdiagnosed who had greater degrees of stenosis than was revealed by the DSA.

The results of the study indicated that, in the cases where there was good visualization of the renal arteries, the accuracy of DSA compared to aortography was 95%.

Abdominal aortic pathology has been accurately diagnosed in 40 patients when compared to the results of surgery and abdominal aortography. These diagnoses included occlusion, intraluminal clots, aneurysm, and aortic dissection which were readily identified.

The peripheral circulation in the iliac and femoral arteries can be adequately identified with intravenous DSA for the detection of occlusive disease, aneurysms, and vascular grafting procedures (Fig. 2). Diagnostic studies have been obtained in vessels as far distal as the foot. The extent of the examination is limited to the size of the image-intensifier input diameter so that when the entire extremity needs to be studied, multiple injections must be made.

Sequential studies of the lower extremities, using a programmable moving table, with multiple masks being made prior to the injection of contrast material and later reregistration may in the future extend the use of DSA for peripheral angiography.

Enhanced visualization of the arteries of the foot by DSA after intra-aortic injections have been demonstrated in several patients when catheter angiography gave inconclusive results using film as a detector.

Similarly, intravenous DSA studies of the upper extremity have given visualization equivalent to that of catheter angiography of the arm vessels in a few patients. However, identification of arteries of the hand has required intra-arterial injections into the brachial artery, magnification techniques, and a matrix with the smallest pixel size available.

3.6 Selective Catheter Intra-arterial Studies

Digital subtraction angiography may be used instead of film as a receptor for intra-arterial catheterization studies. While a systematic analysis has not been carried out, examples of tumor staining in the hepatic and renal circulation have been revealed by DSA when they have not been revealed by film subtraction techniques.

4 Special Applications

Availability of digital storage permits a wide range of programming for assessment of physiologic events contained in the serial anatomic images. The numerical information contained in each pixel from the serial images can be utilized for temporal study of the iodine signal using region-of-interest cursors. In addition, parametric images such as time-to-maximum concentration of contrast material in each pixel can be used to create a single composite image reflecting contrast material arrival and transit (*Gallagher* et al., to be published). Images obtained using EKG gating permit application of programs to measure ejection fraction of the left ventricle. Two inherent potential inaccuracies in quantitation of the iodine signal, Compton scatter and veiling glare, can also be corrected in software to increase the accuracy of the measurements.

Graphs of the concentration of radiographic contrast material as a function of time are useful measurements of the function in the organ or blood vessel of interest. However, these graphs represent an average function of some region which has been selected for analysis. An alternative method for analysis is a composite image of the entire area or organ.

The parametric image serves the need of creating a picture which can represent some parameter of the time/concentration curve in each pixel. From a timed sequence of images, the concentration of contrast material as a function of location and time, $C(x, y, t)$ may be used to derive a parametric image as a function of location, $P(x, y)$. This derived parameter may represent a slope, a rate constant, an extremal value, a time of occurrence, etc (*Gallagher* et al., to be published).

In our preprototype unit, images were converted to a storage format in which images were stored as frames rather than difference frames. Hence, the pixel values

(DSA numbers) are proportional to the logarithm of the signal intensity at that point. Thus, the DSA value at a pixel point, x, y, is

$$DSA\ (x, y) = C_1\ \ln\ (I_0\ (x, y)\ \exp\ (- u\ dz) + CS + VG) + C_2$$

where C_1 and C_2 are the gain and bias of the logarithmic amplifier, I_0 is the incident x-ray intensity, u and z the linear attenuation coefficient of and the path length through the imaged object, CS the term due to Compton scattering, and VG the contribution of veiling glare in the imaging system. The dependence of the x-ray energy which is quite important and complex has been suppressed for simplicity. Changes in the concentration of the radiographic contrast material are reflected as changes in the linear attenuation coefficient and changes in the DSA numbers. As long as the variation in Compton scattering and veiling glare are small compared to variation in the directly attenuated intensity term, the critical points of the curve of DSA values as a function of time occur at the same time as the critical points of the concentration as a function of time. Such a result can be shown by the differentiation of the equation above. Thus, a peaking concentration of radiographic contrast material occurs at a minimum in the DSA values.

5 Practical Problems

Two major problems limit the consistency in the quality of DSA images. The first consists of misregistration due to gross or subtle patient motion occurring between the selected mask frame and the contrast frame. The second is the inherent limitation resulting from global injection of contrast material where vessels of interest are obscured by other regional vessels which overlap them.

Even with the advantage of rapid remasking to produce subtraction images where the mask is temporally as close to the arrival of contrast material as possible, motion artifacts can produce severe problems. Patient swallowing in the study of the extracranial carotid circulation produces gross misregistration artifacts. No satisfactory method has been defined to date to alleviate this problem without the necessity for producing complications such as reaction to topical anesthesia. In the abdomen, intestinal peristalsis is the primary cause of misregistration artifacts. Intravenous administration of 2 mg glucagon assists in decresing the number of these artifacts, but in some patients, even at this dose level, peristaltic motion still occurs. This represents a particular problem in imaging of organs such as the kidney, where the slightest misregistration artifact will obscure the smaller vessels in the kidney at the segmental or arcuate levels.

In addition to the two limitations discussed above, the field size of the image intensifier also produces a limitation in certain areas of the body. The extremities are the primary example where the field coverage of the image intensifier would require three to four injections of contrast material to adequately view the entire extremity. While this does not represent a serious problem in the study of a single extremity, the usual patient with arteriosclerosis obliterans is likely to have the disease in both legs, and it would not appear to be safe to make all of the injections · required to visualize both extremities in a single patient examination.

An additional problem relates to the high contrast sensitivity of the system, an advantage in most areas, but disadvantageous in certain regions such as the lung. The enormous number of pulmonary arteries at the third order and smaller size, integrated along the beam projection, tend to obscure one another.

Cardiac motion has not proven to be as serious a limitation as was originally thought. At framing rates of six per second and at frame exposure times of 5–15 ms, good anatomic images can be obtained. For certain applications, images obtained with EKG gating have proven useful in ascertaining the phase of the cardiac cycle in which the images were obtained. For patients with intracardiac shunts, particularly atrial septal defects, very high framing rates may not uncover the shunt. However, region of interest cursors placed over the right atrium permit the detection of recirculation of contrast material.

6 Cost/Benefit Evaluation

Cost/benefit analyses on digital subtraction angiography have not been carried out in a systematic manner. Our clinical experience to date suggests that for the standard clinical indications for angiography, the availability of DSA will significantly reduce the need for conventional angiography with its associated costs for the procedure and for hospitalization. At the Cleveland Clinic Foundation, total patient charges for DSA, carried out on an outpatient basis, are only 15% of the costs which would be incurred for a conventional angiogram on a patient hospitalized for 1 day. Additional savings to the health care system should be anticipated because of the relative complication-free digital subtraction angiography as compared with, for example, a stroke sequela to a conventional carotid angiogram. Such savings are difficult, if not impossible, to quantify but are, nonetheless, real.

On the other hand, the ease and simplicity of digital subtraction angiography has resulted in DSA studies being carried out on patients for indications that would usually not prompt a conventional angiogram. Two major examples are studies of the extracranial cerebral circulation in patients with asymptomatic carotid bruits and evaluation of postoperative bypass grafts carried out on a routine basis to serve as a baseline for such patients who ultimately will return with progressive arteriosclerosis obliterans. In addition, patients with asymptomatic carotid bruits, who are found to have moderate occlusive disease, will most likely prompt a conventional angiogram and perhaps surgery, which would not have been carried out if the patient had not been evaluated by DSA. Offsetting these costs would be the potential of stroke prevention and its savings to the health care system in terms of rehabilitation costs and lost worker productivity.

References

Brennecke R, Brown TK, Bursch J et al. (1977) Computerized videoimage processing with application to cardioangiographic roentgen image series. In: Nagel HH (ed) Digital image processing. Springer, Berlin Heidelberg New York, p 244

Buonocore E, Meaney TF, Borkowski GP et al. (1981) Digital subtraction angiography of the abdominal aorta and renal arteries. Radiology 139:281–286

Chilcote WA, Modic MT, Pavlicek WA et al. (1981) Digital subtraction angiography of the carotid arteries: a comparative study in 100 patients. Radiology 139:287–295

Christenson PC, Ovitt TW, Fisher HD et al. (1980) Intravenous angiography using digital video subtraction: intravenous cervicocerebrovascular angiography. Am J Neuroradiol 1:379–386

Crummy AB, Strother CM, Sackett JF et al. (1980) Computerized fluoroscopy: Digital subtraction for intravenous angiocardiography and arteriography. AJR 135:1131–1140

Ergun EL, Mistretta CA, Kruger RA et al. (1979) A hybrid computerized fluoroscopy technique for noninvasive cardiovascular imaging. Radiology 132:739–742

Gallagher JH, Meaney TF, Flechner SM et al. (to be published) Parametric imaging of digital subtraction angiography studies for renal transplant evaluation

Hillman BJ, Ovitt TW, Nudelman S et al. (1981) Digital video subtraction angiography of renal vascular abnormalities. Radiology 139:277–280

Kruger RA, Mistretta CA, Houk TL et al. (1979a) Computerized fluoroscopy in real time for noninvasive visualization of the cardiovascular system. Preliminary studies. Radiology 130:49–57

Kruger RA, Mistretta CA, Houk TL et al. (1979b) Computerized fluoroscopy techniques for noninvasive study of cardiac chamber dynamics. Invest Radiol 14:279–287

Meaney TF, Weinstein MA, Buonocore E, et al. (1980a) Digital subtraction angiography of the human cardiovascular system. SPIE 233:272–278

Meaney TF, Weinstein MA, Buonocore E et al. (1980b) Digital subtraction angiography of the human cardiovascular system. AJR 135:1153–1160

Modic MT, Weinstein MA, Chilcote WA et al. (to be published) DSA of the intracranial vascular system: a comparative study in 55 patients. AJNR

Ovitt TW, Capp MP, Fisher HD et al. (1978) The development of a digital video subtraction system for intravenous angiography. In: Miller HA, Schmidt EV, Harrison PC (eds) Noninvasive cardiovascular measurements, vol 167. Society of Photo-Optical Instrumentation Engineers, Bellingham, Washington, pp 61–65

Ovitt T, Capp MP, Christenson P et al. (1979) Development of a digital video subtraction system for intravenous angiography. SPIE 206:73

Ovitt TW, Christenson PC, Fisher HD et al. (1980) Intravenous angiography using digital video subtraction: x-ray imaging system. AJNR 1:387–390

Strother CM, Sackett JF, Crummy AB et al. (1980) Clinical applications of computerized fluoroscopy. The extracranial carotid arteries. Radiology 136:781–783

References for Further Reading on Nuclear Magnetic Resonance

Brownell GL, Budinger TF, Lauterbur PC, McGeer PL (1982) Positron tomography and nuclear magnetic resonance imaging. Science 215:619–626

Budinger TF (1981) Nuclear magnetic resonance (NMR) in vivo studies: known thresholds for health effects. J Com Ass Tomogr 5:800–811

Doyle FH, Pennock JM, Banks LM, McDonnell MJ, Bydder GM, Steiner RE, Young IR, Clarke GJ, Pasmore T, Gilderdale DJ (1982) Nuclear magnetic resonance imaging of the liver: initial experience. AJR 138:193–200

Doyle FH, Pennock JM, Orr JS, Gore JC, Bydder GM, Steiner RE (1981) Imaging of the brain by nuclear magnetic resonance. Lancet 8237:53–57

Epstein FH (1981) Nuclear magnetic resonance. A new tool in clinical medicine. N Engl J Med. 304:1360–1361

Gadian DG (1982) Nuclear magnetic resonance and its applications to living systems. Clarendon Press, Oxford.

James AE, Partain CL, Holland GN, Gore JC, Rollo FD, Harms SE, Price RR (1981) Nuclear magnetic resonance imaging: the current state. AJR 138:201–210

Mallard J (1981) The noes have it! Do they? Brit J Radiol 54:831–849

Smith FW, Reid A, Hutchison JMS, Mallard JR (1982) Nuclear magnetic resonance: imaging of the pancreas. Radiology 142:677–680

Young IR, Burl M, Clarke GJ, Hall AS, Pasmore T, Collins AG, Smith DT, Orr JS, Bydder GM, Doyle FH, Greenspan RH, Steiner RE (1981) Magnetic resonance properties of hydrogen imaging the posterior fossa. AJR 137:895–901

Young IR, Bailes DR, Burl M, Collins AG, Smith DT, McDonnell MJ, Orr JS, Banks LM, Bydder GM, Greenspan RH, Steiner RE (1982) Initial clinical evaluation of the whole body nuclear magnetic resonance (NMR) tomograph. J Com Ass Tomogr 6:1–18

Frontiers in European Radiology

Editors-in-Chief:
A.L. Baert, E. Boijsen,
W.A. Fuchs, F.H.W. Heuck

aims – to provide a platform for European radiological research
– to strengthen the position of radiology in clinical medicine by integrating the various approaches to clinical and experimental radiology

Frontiers in European Radiology (FER) addresses radiologists all over the world with the goal of improving the international exchange of information on all aspects of radiological research. This exchange has unfortunately been limited in the past, especially by the language barriers involved. As a result, Europe's contribution to scientific progress in this interdisciplinary specialty has influenced only regional developments. A first step toward rectifying the situation was taken in Hamburg in September 1979, when the formation of the association of European University Radiologists was discussed and decided upon.
FER is the logical continuation of that initiative; it will provide a forum for scientists in European clinical and experimental radiology where important reports on progress in the field can be presented in a depth not possible in a journal. It will be a concise source of detailed information for those wanting to keep abreast of the scientific progress in this field.

Volume 1

1982. 113 figures in 187 separate illustrations.
V, 170 pages. ISBN 3-540-10753-3

Contents:
I. Fernström, B. Johansson: Percutaneous Extraction of Renal Calculi. – *R. Günther, P. Alken:* Percutaneous Nephropyelostomy and Endo-Urological Manipulations. – *R. Pasariello, G. P. Feltrin, D. Miotto, S. Pedrazzoli, P. Rossi, G. Simonetti:* Transhepatic Portal Catheterization with Pancreatic Venous Sampling Versus Angiography in the Localization of Pancreatic Functioning Tumors. – *G. M. Kauffmann, G. Richter, J. Rassweiler, R. Rohrbach:* New Topics in Embolization. Effects of Central, Peripheral or Capillary Occlusion Type in Animal Models Simulating Tumor Embolization. – *F. Brunelle:* Electric Transcatheter Vascular Obliteration: Electrothrombosis. Electrolysis or Electrocoagulation. – *V. Hegedüs, O. Winding, J. Grønvall, P. Faarup:* Manufacturing-Derived Impurities in Angiography. – *K.-H. Hübener:* Digital Radiography Using a Computed Tomography Instrument

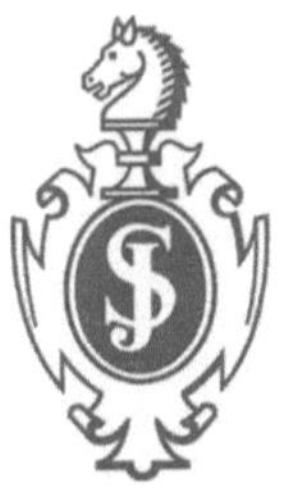

Springer-Verlag
Berlin
Heidelberg
New York

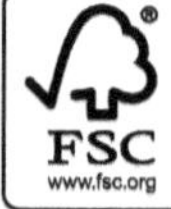